To Shan...

INFORMATION
IS THE BEST
MEDICINE

A Guide to Navigating
Your Healthcare

Be well...

Peace,

GL

GLENN ELLIS

1-28-18

Information is the Best Medicine

Copyright 2012, Glenn Ellis

www.glennellis.com

ISBN: 978-0-615-55767-0

The Jewel in the Robe

There once was a man who had a rich friend. One day the man called on his friend who entertained him until, sated on wine, he fell asleep. The rich friend was called away on business. Before leaving, as a parting gift he sewed a priceless jewel into the hem of the sleeping man's garment. Knowing nothing of this, the man awoke and went about his business. Falling on hard times, he wandered the world in poverty. Years later, they met again. The rich man, astonished at his friend's condition, told him of the gift he had given him, and which he had possessed all along.

- The Lotus Sutra -

This book is lovingly dedicated to the memory
of my departed siblings:

Randolph Ellis, Jr.
Irma Ellis Patterson
Edwin Dotson Ellis, Sr.

ACKNOWLEDGEMENTS

With deepest gratitude and respect, I must thank all those whose have touched my life, and been a source of support, commitment and hope, that have made the work behind this book possible.

No one walks alone and when one is walking on the journey of life just where do you start to thank those that joined you, walked beside you, and helped you along the way.

Much of what I have learned over the years came as the result of being raised by two incredible parents, Hattie Bernice and Randolph Ellis, Sr.

A little bit of each of them will be found here weaving in and out of the pages.

I also have to thank Hilary Beard, with whom I have had the pleasure of working with, and whose words, talent and friendship, over the years has taught me much about my self and the mysterious ways of life.

My thanks to a wonderful man who changed me completely–Dr. Edward S. Cooper, who taught me greater humility, and how to value the lives, thoughts and expressions of others, and how to advocate for, care for, and understand their needs. He has solely made me a more responsible health writer.

Deepest appreciation for my mentor in life, Dr. Daisaku Ikeda, and the Soka Gakkai International, an amazing organization to which I now dedicate much of my life. It is through their teachings, encouragement and support that I have gained and grown. Through this book and my work, throughout my travels, I will continue to spread their message of support to others wishing to develop as human beings.

I owe a tremendous debt of gratitude to Jasmine and Glenn Ellis, Jr., my beloved children, who gave me the inspiration to manifest my potential.

In no particular order, my sincere appreciation goes to: Dr. Lucille W. Ijoy; Bill and Barbara Wilson; Dan Hilferty; Patrick Brown; Barbara Cromartie; María de los Angeles Reyes Figueroa; Kirk Dorn; Nadine Bonner; Cheryl Dickerson; Michael Rashid; Fatimah and Kenny Gamble; Marie K. and Robert W. Bogle; Dr. Arlene Ackerman; Mercer Redcross, Jillian M. Oliver; George Curry; Dr. Mark G. Kuczewski; Linda Vitali; Mrs. Lottie Palmer; Abdur Rahim Islam; Dr. Kayhan P. Parsi; Susan L. Taylor; Lee Bailey; Dr. Arnold Eiser; Terrie Williams; Lisa Hoggs; Patty Jackson; Dominique DiPrima; Sonia Sanchez; Dr. David Nash; Sonny Hill; Milton Perry; Suran Casselle; Barbara Grant; Rubin Benson; Bill Lucy; Anita Patterson; Lillian and Dick Gregory; Sharon Silver; Cody Anderson; Janet S. Lynch; Mrs. Verdell Odom; Stevie Wonder; Leon and Carol Ware; Father Peter Clark; Clarence Edwards; Deborah Bolling; Dr. J. Bruce Smith; Lila Williams; Father and Mrs. Thomas Logan; Charlene Horne; Dr. Walter and Beverly Lomax; Deni Hagains-Goss; Jerry Mondesire; and countless others,

Acknowledgements

for whom space will not permit me to name individually, but whose contribution was no less valuable.

I am eternally grateful for Dr. Hattie Bryant Witt-Greene, my Brunetta C. Hill Elementary School library teacher, who taught me to use the library -the most liberating moment of my life. Also, to my English teacher at A. H. Parker High School in Birmingham, Mr. Theodore Roosevelt Hawkins, who helped begin my love affair with words and writing.

Sadly they have both passed on, so my thanks to their families, and all those who loved them as much as I did.

Many of you have continuously urged me to write another book–to share my insights, together with an informed, positive approach to the myriad of health issues that life throws at us.

Perhaps this book and it's pages will be seen as "thanks" to the tens of thousands of you who have helped make my life journey what is today.

So at last, here it is.

Glenn Ellis
January, 2012

TABLE OF CONTENTS

TABLE OF CONTENTS *(Continued)*

PREFACE

───────

Many years ago, as a Pre-Medical student, I had an experience that, as I look back, changed my life forever!

Little did I know, that more than any course I enrolled in, or any other of my educational experiences up to that point, this usually normal encounter would result in my life being thrust on a path that I would continue on until this very day.

An African American medical doctor, who was doing his residency at Philadelphia General Hospital, stopped by my apartment, as he would often do throughout my undergraduate years. He had functioned as a mentor to me, as I was trying desperately to find my way through the maze of the challenging curriculum required to prepare me for my lifelong dream: going to medical school!

But it all came to an abrupt halt that hot, humid summer day in Philadelphia.

My friend told me that on that day, he had to take a patient he was caring for (a 35-year-old African American man) off of life support. His words and the look deep in his eyes conveyed a feeling of fear that left me paralyzed.

I had dreamed of becoming a doctor, and taking care of the precious lives that had been a part of my warm childhood memories, and who had protected me from being scarred by the horors of the civl rights movement of the 1960's. I felt it was my obligation to be a doctor. I had the best teachers, preachers, leaders, family, you name it. They all made a contribution in preparing me for the journey.

But there I was, in Philadelphia taking summer college courses, sitting on the couch in my apartment with my mouth dropped open, unable to move after what I had just heard: A man was allowed to die when my friend removed him from life support, because his "higher ups" had determined it was futile to continue care.

Following that day, two questions were raised that would set off a course of events, which in me no longer playing an active role in the direction my life would take: 1) was I not mature enough to handle having that much control over another human beings' life; and 2) what could have happened in only 35 years that a man could end up in such a dismal state of health?

As it turned out, the first question paled in comparision to the enlightenment and sense of purpose and clarity from the second question.

As I pondered these questions over the next few years, trying to "find myself", I came to understand the concept of "Social Determinants of Health".

The social determinants of health are the conditions in which people are born, grow and are educated, live, work and age, including the health system. These circumstances are shaped by the distribution of money, power and resources at global, national and local levels, which are themselves influenced by policy choices. These social determinants of health are mostly responsible for health inequities–the unfair and avoidable differences in health status seen within and between people and even between countries.

I came to understand why a 35-year-old man could end up with such a fate. I could see clearly how so many doctors face making the same scenario that my friend faced.

Out of it all, I came to realize that health is a lot like my personal experience with credit: by the time I realized what it was; what was required to protect and take care of it; and how valuable it was to impacting the quality of life...I had destroyed it! I just didn't know better. You see, like credit, many of us are driven to make consumer decisions without understanding the true "cost" of our decisions.

So, my life has been one of being devoted to improving the information available to people so that they are capable of making "informed decisions" about matters of health. I'm convinced that the 35-year-old man did make some lifestyle, diet, and/or behavior choices that landed him in that bed at Philadelphia General Hospital, based on not having good information.

Information is the Best Medicine

It was clear that in order to focus attention on the social determinants of health, it is important to understand how these social determinants of health come to influence health and cause disease. For millions of people in America, these health-threatening behaviors are a response to material deprivation and stress. Social environments determine whether individuals take up tobacco, use alcohol, experience poor diets, and have low levels of physical activity. Tobacco and excessive alcohol use, and carbohydrate-dense diets are also means of coping with difficult circumstances.

My intention with this book is to provide some insight and understanding to many areas and topics which most of us will find touching our lives, either directly or indirectly. The benefits of this knowledge include improved communication with your doctors, greater adherence to treatment, greater ability to engage in self-care, improved health status, and healthier lifestyle and diet choices for you and your family.

Over the 15 years that I have written a weekly column to this end, I have covered a range of very critical subjects, which have made a difference to many. Taking a look back at this body of writing, I bring to you the most effective "prescription" you will ever receive. As you will hopefully discover, in spite of the United States having the most expensive healthcare system in the world, you will find that, **"Information is the Best Medicine"**.

Live the best Life possible!

Peace,

Glenn Ellis Sr.

ARE YOU SICK OR JUST AGING?

Pharmaceutical companies in the United States spend a huge, huge amount of money annually on commercial advertising. Many drug companies have found that they can readily and easily increase their revenue streams by appealing directly to the consumer through television drug commercials. Rather than rely solely on physicians recommending one med over another, these companies are reaching out directly to the end-use consumer through television drug commercials.

As we all know, most people see a TV commercial, and are quickly convinced that they must need the advertised medication for their "condition".

Unfortunately, this is, in many cases, the result of us having no understanding of what happens when the body ages.

Normal signs of aging are generally the same for everyone, though they don't necessarily develop at a particular age. You can expect to notice and adjust to, many gradual changes as you age. Certain physical changes are fairly predictable. Most people start needing reading glasses between ages 40 and 50, and many have some hearing loss later in life.

As people age, bones tend to become less dense. Thus, bones become weaker and more likely to break. In women, loss of bone density speeds up after menopause.

Bones become less dense partly because the amount of calcium they contain decreases. Part of the reason is that less calcium is absorbed in the digestive tract and levels of vitamin D (which helps the body use calcium) decrease slightly. Calcium is the main mineral that gives bones strength. Certain bones are weakened more than others. Those most affected include the end of the thighbone (femur) at the hip, the ends of the arm bones at the wrist, and the bones of the spine.

Ligaments, which bind joints together, tend to become less elastic as people age, making joints feel tight or stiff. This change results from chemical changes in the proteins that make up the ligaments. Consequently, most people become less flexible as they age. Ligaments also will tend to tear more easily, and when they tear, they heal more slowly.

Aging affects the digestive system in several ways. Food is emptied from the stomach more slowly, and the stomach cannot hold as much food because it is less elastic. But in most people, these changes are too slight to be noticed.

Certain changes in the digestive system do cause problems in some people. The digestive tract may produce less lactase; an enzyme the body needs to digest milk. As a result, older people are more likely to develop intolerance of dairy products. In some people, this slowing may contribute to constipation.

The liver also changes. It tends to become smaller, and less blood flows through it. As a result, the liver may be slightly less able to help rid the body of drugs and other substances. And the effects of drugs last longer.

As people age, the kidneys tend to become smaller, and less blood flows through them. Beginning at about age 30, the kidneys begin to filter blood less well. As years pass, they may remove waste products from the blood less well. They may also excrete too much water, making dehydration more likely.

The urinary tract changes in several ways that may make controlling urination more difficult. The maximum amount of urine that the bladder can hold decreases. As you get older you may be less able to delay urination after the first sense of a need to urinate. The bladder muscles weaken. As a result, more urine is left in the bladder after urination is finished. These changes are one reason that urinary incontinence (the uncontrollable loss of urine) becomes more common as people age.

As women age, the urethra (which carries urine out of the body) shortens and its lining becomes thinner. The muscle that controls the passage of urine through the urethra (urinary sphincter) is less able to close tightly and prevent leakage. These changes may result from the decrease in the estrogen level that occurs with menopause.

As men age, the prostate gland tends to enlarge. In many men, it enlarges enough to partly block the passage of urine.

As people age, the heart and blood vessels change in many ways. The walls of the heart become stiffer, and the heart fills with blood more slowly.

In aging men, owing to the decreasing testosterone levels, there is reduced interest for intimacy and diminished drive for any form of sexual activities. Similarly, in aging women, owing to the reduced estrogen levels, there is a phenomenal change in their behavior, needs, and desires for intimacy after menopause.

The walls of the arteries become thicker and less elastic. The arteries become less able to respond to changes in the amount of blood pumped through them. Thus, blood pressure is higher in older people than in younger people.

Despite these changes, a normal older heart functions well. At rest, the differences between young and old hearts are small. The differences become apparent only when more work is required of the heart, as occurs when a person exercises vigorously or becomes sick. An older heart cannot increase how fast it beats as quickly or as much as a younger heart. Regular exercise can reduce many of the effects of aging on the heart and blood vessels.

The muscles used in breathing, such as the diaphragm, tend to weaken. Also, slightly less oxygen is absorbed from air that is breathed in. In people who do not smoke or have a lung disorder, the muscles of breathing and the lungs continue to function well enough to meet the needs of the body during ordinary daily activities. But these changes may make exercising vigorously (for example, running or biking energetically) more difficult. The lungs become less able to fight infection, in part because the cells that sweep debris out of the airways are less able to do so. Coughing, which also helps clear the lungs, tends to be weaker.

Most vital organs gradually become less efficient with age. Your metabolism gradually slows, which means that your body needs less food energy than before. The kidneys also become less able to keep your body hydrated. This makes exercise, water intake, and a well-balanced diet increasingly important over time. An active body that gets plenty of oxygen, water, and nutrients is more likely to function efficiently for a longer period of time.

As my Grandpapa, John Roberts, would say, "this only happens if you live long enough".

IS IT IMPOSSIBLE TO BE
HEALTHY IN AMERICA?

Health literacy – the ability to read, understand
and act on health information

Research shows that most consumers need help understanding
health care information; regardless of reading level, patients prefer medical information that is easy to read and understand. For people
who don't have strong reading skills, however, easy-to-read health care
materials are essential.

The health of 90 million people in the U.S. may be at risk because
of the difficulty some patients experience in understanding and acting
upon health information.

One out of five American adults reads at the 5th grade level or
below, and the average American reads at the 8th to 9th grade level, yet
most health care materials are written above the 10th grade level.

Limited health literacy increases the disparity in health care access among exceptionally vulnerable populations (such as racial/ethnic minorities and the elderly).

According to the Center for Health Care Strategies, a disproportionate number of minorities and immigrants are estimated to have literacy problems:

- 50% of Hispanics
- 40% of Blacks
- 33% of Asians

In fact, more than 66% of US adults age 60 and over have either inadequate or marginal literacy skills, and 50% of welfare recipients read below fifth grade level!

So, imagine what this means in major urban cities around this country where the populations are mostly brown and black people.

Never mind that all of these cities have world-class medical centers, hospitals, and the latest in pharmaceuticals and treatments. They mean nothing to people who are disproportionately sicker, poorer, and uneducated. How is it possible for them to benefit?

And it's not just these poor souls who suffer. Low health literacy is an enormous cost burden on the American healthcare system – annual health care costs for individuals with low literacy skills are *4 times higher* than those with higher literacy skills.

Even problems with patient compliance and medical errors may be based on poor understanding of health care information. Only about 50% of all patients take medications as directed.

Patients with low health literacy and chronic diseases, such as diabetes, asthma, or hypertension, have less knowledge of their disease and its treatment and fewer correct self-management skills than literate patients. Patients with low literacy skills have a 50% increased risk of hospitalization, compared with patients who had adequate literacy skills.

The research suggests that people with low literacy:

- Make more medication or treatment errors
- Are less able to comply with treatments
- Lack the skills needed to successfully negotiate the health care system
- Are at a higher risk for hospitalization than people with adequate literacy skills

Let's not forget that in the wake of the new national health reform, health systems, health plans, providers, and policy makers are attempting to see what can be done to contain health care costs. For them, it is important to understand that health care spending is not distributed evenly across the population—or by condition. In fact, just five percent of the U.S. population—those with the most complex and extensive medical conditions—accounts for almost half (49 percent) of total U.S. health care spending, and 20 percent of the population accounts for 80 percent of total spending.

In medicine, a chronic disease is a disease that is long lasting or recurrent. The most common chronic conditions are high blood pressure, diabetes, arthritis, high cholesterol, and respiratory diseases like asthma and emphysema. These are the very conditions commonly mentioned when we hear talk of "health disparities", in reference to minorities and people of color.

Is it Impossible to Be Healthy in America?

According to an Institute of Medicine (2004) report, low health literacy negatively affects the treatment outcome and safety of care delivery. The report points out that these patients have a higher risk of hospitalization and longer hospital stays, are less likely to comply with treatment, are more likely to make errors with medication, and are more ill when they seek medical care.

Those with poor health literacy are more likely to have a chronic disease and less likely to get the health care they need. Individuals with inadequate functional health literacy often struggle with basic tasks when managing a chronic condition such as reading and comprehending prescription bottles, appointment slips, self-management instructions, and educational brochures. Inadequate functional health literacy can be a barrier to controlling disease and can subsequently lead to poor health outcomes and increased health care costs.

Chronic conditions are the leading cause of death and disability in the U.S. and treating patients with comorbid chronic conditions costs up to seven times as much as treating patients who have only one chronic condition. Modifiable health risk factors, such as cigarette smoking and overweight/obesity, are responsible for much of the illness, healthcare utilization, and subsequent costs related to chronic disease.

Reading abilities are typically three to five grade levels below the last year of school completed. Therefore, people with a high school diploma, typically read at a seventh or eighth grade reading level.

Every school day, more than 7,200 students fall through the cracks of America's public high schools. Three out of every 10 members of this year's graduating class, 1.3 million students in all, will fail to graduate with a diploma. The effects of this graduation crisis fall disproportionately on the nation's most vulnerable youths and communities. A majority of non-graduates are members of historically disadvantaged minorities and other educationally underserved groups. They are more likely to attend school in large, urban districts. And they come disproportionately from communities challenged by severe poverty and economic hardship.

The average adult in the United States reads at an eighth-grade level yet most patient education materials are written on a high school or college reading level!

In case you haven't noticed, I am deeply saddened by the countless, helpless millions all over this country who don't stand a chance.

Over the years, I have become absolutely convinced of the intersection between health and basic education, and I have witnessed countless horror stories to prove it.

Hospitalizations; Clinical Trials; Medication Errors; Unhealthy Behaviors...just to name a few.

Yes, America, we should all be ashamed.

Regardless of how we have allowed our health and public education systems to degenerate, the fact remains that all of us deserve to enjoy the ability to be healthy and to be educated. It's not a privilege, it's a right!

As we consider how to "reset" the Health Reform Act, and "reform" our public education system, we need to look at what we have become as a society.

Here's another word definition:

Is it Impossible to Be Healthy in America?

Degenerate–Having lost the physical, mental, or moral qualities considered normal and desirable; showing evidence of decline

While pondering this, let me leave you with this:

"The most certain test by which we judge whether a country is really free is the amount of security enjoyed by minorities"

- JOHN E. E. DALBERG, Lord Acton,
The History of Freedom in Antiquity, 1877 -

HUNGER

=====

We've all seen news reports about people who are starving in countries plagued by war or drought. Unfortunately, many people in the world go hungry because they can't get enough to eat most of the time.

According to a new report by the U.S. Department of Agriculture, 17.4 million American families–almost 15 percent of U.S. households– are now "food insecure," an almost 30 percent increase since 2006. This means that, during any given month, they will be out of money, out of food, and forced to miss meals or seek assistance to feed themselves.

The nation's economic crisis has catapulted the number of Americans who lack enough food to the highest level since the government has been keeping track, according to a new federal report, which shows that nearly 50 million people — including almost one child in four — struggled last year to get enough to eat.

I myself have recently broadened my focus to the plight of the thousands of Somali's who are dying everyday as a result of politics and the monumental drought in Eastern Africa. Seeing hundreds of babies die daily from starvation is something I certainly can't ignore.

But don't be mistaken; this is not only happening in some far away land. Philadelphia ranks near the top of our nation's hunger list, for the second year in a row!

The consequences of having such a poor and hungry place in its midst can be catastrophic for a city, whose young people risk being developmentally compromised by a dearth of nutritious food in their first years.

Hunger is the most commonly used term to describe the social condition of people (or organisms) who frequently experience, or live with the threat of experiencing, the physical sensation of desiring food.

We all feel hungry at times. Hunger is the way the body signals that it needs to eat. Once we're able to eat enough food to satisfy our body's needs, we stop being hungry. Teens can feel hungry a lot because their rapidly growing and developing bodies demand extra food.

People with malnutrition lack the nutrients necessary for their bodies to grow and stay healthy. Someone can be malnourished for a long or short period of time, and the condition may be mild or severe. Malnutrition can affect someone's physical and mental health. People who are suffering from malnutrition are more likely to get sick; in very severe cases, they may even die from its effects.

We live in the world's wealthiest nation. Yet, 13 percent of people living in the United States live in poverty. In many ways, America is the land of plenty. But for 1 in 6 Americans, hunger is a reality. Many people believe that the problems associated with hunger are confined to small pockets of society, certain areas of the country, or certain neighborhoods, but the reality is much different.

Right now, millions of Americans are struggling with hunger. We all know and are in contact with people affected by hunger, even though we might not be aware of it.

Philadelphia has one of the highest child poverty rates in the US—one child out of three lives at or below the federal poverty level. Many young children and their parents are at risk for food insecurity and hunger.

It also has the highest poverty rate of any major U.S. city, with one out of four people living in poverty. One-third of that population is under 18.

The truth of the matter is that certain groups experience food insecurity at far higher rates than the rest of the U.S. population. According to USDA, the rate of household and child "food insecurity" among African-Americans and Hispanics is more than twice as high as that of whites.

Why don't they just make healthier choices with what little food they have you say?

Even when the poor do attempt to eat healthy, it hurts us. A study published earlier this year in the American Journal of Preventive Medicine showed that so-called "fresh" fruits and vegetables and ground beef found in poor neighborhood groceries were more likely to be covered in bacteria and have higher mold and contaminant counts than those found in wealthier areas. In fact, people who have plenty to eat may still be malnourished if they don't eat food that provides the right nutrients, vitamins, and minerals.

A nutritious diet can help one climb out of poverty or homelessness, but poverty (and homelessness) makes it nearly impossible to maintain a nutritious diet. While some of the rich and skinny continue to condemn low-income Americans for being obese, I challenge them to come up a plan for eating healthy on $15 a week. I'd also like to see them design a menu that a single mother working two or three jobs can fix in four to eight minutes!

To better understand the senselessness of this madness, here are some surprising facts about the food supply in America:

- **40-50% of all food ready for harvest never gets eaten.** Research done by a professor at the University of Arizona has shown that nearly half the food produced in the United States every year goes to waste. While news of our throw-away society isn't necessarily surprising, that so much of what we produce is wasted while millions in our own nation and those around the world go hungry should be appalling.
- **Every year, over 25% of Americans get sick from what they eat.** This means some 76 million food borne infections, 350,000 of which require hospitalization and 5,000 of which are deadly. Think your food is safe?
- **As few as 13 major corporations control nearly all of the slaughterhouses in the U.S.** Why should you care? Because these major corporations pack a lot of political power, making them incredibly difficult to regulate and inspect.
- **Americans eat 31% more packaged food than fresh food.** This means that Americans eat more packaged and processed food than people in any other country, according to the New York Times. Packaged foods themselves aren't necessarily bad

for us, but Americans tend to consume frozen pizzas and microwave dinners, which can be high in fats and salts.

- **A simple frozen dinner can contains ingredients from over 500 different suppliers.** NPR has shown that a basic frozen prepared meal can contain up to 50 different ingredients. These ingredients come from all over the world, changing hands numerous times along the way. This means that in order to trust that your food is safe; you have to trust that all of those hundreds of companies along the way stuck to regulations about food safety.

- **50% of tested samples of high fructose corn syrup tested for mercury.** There has been a lot of debate about the safety and health of high fructose corn syrup lately, and some believe with pretty good reason. HFCS is found in a wide range of food products from bread to catsup.

- **Americans eat about six to nine pounds of chemical food additives per year.** While it may seem that the amount of chemicals you're eating in your food is inconsequential, over the year they add up. Some may be harmless to you, but others may have effects that are yet unknown over a long period of time.

- **Food intolerance is on the rise, with as many as 30 million people in the U.S. showing symptoms.** Some believe that the growth in food allergies and food intolerance may have to do with our diets. Eating yeast-based foods, preserved meats and processed foods can lead to greater levels of histamine in the body which many people are incapable of processing naturally.

- **Fewer than 27% of Americans eat the correct ratio of meats**

to vegetables. Studies have shown that eating too much meat increases your cancer risk, a fact reinforced by the longer life span of cultures that focus more heavily on veggies than meats. By not eating enough of these vegetables, many Americans are missing out on the healthy nutrients, minerals and compounds they contain.

If only poor people understood nutrition, and could do something about it...

THERE'S NO "ALTERNATIVE" TO MEDICINE

In response to a recent series of radio health tips I did, I have been receiving a number of "unfavorable" comments from friends and fans alike.

It seems that (due in large part to my background in Herbal Medicine and Homeopathy), interpret the suggestions I often make, which speak about seeing medical doctors and taking prescription drugs, as a form of "betrayal".

People have used herbal medicines throughout history and they are currently the most commonly used medicines worldwide.

Many Americans use complementary and alternative medicine (CAM) in pursuit of health and well-being. The 2007 National Health Interview Survey (NHIS), which included a comprehensive survey of CAM use by Americans, showed that approximately 38 percent of adults use CAM.

There's No "Alternative" to Medicine

Defining CAM is difficult, because the field is very broad and constantly changing. National Center for Complementary and Alternative Medicine (NCCAM) defines CAM as a group of diverse medical and health care systems, practices, and products that are not generally considered part of conventional medicine. Conventional medicine (also called Western or allopathic medicine) is medicine as practiced by holders of M.D. (medical doctor) and D.O. (doctor of osteopathic medicine;) degrees and by allied health professionals, such as physical therapists, psychologists, and registered nurses. The boundaries between CAM and conventional medicine are not absolute, and specific CAM practices may, over time, become widely accepted.

"Complementary medicine" refers to use of CAM **together with** conventional medicine, such as using acupuncture in addition to usual care to help lessen pain. Most use of CAM by Americans is complementary. "Alternative medicine" refers to use of CAM **in place of** conventional medicine. "Integrative medicine" (also called integrated medicine) refers to a practice that combines both conventional and CAM treatments for which there is evidence of safety and effectiveness.

We've all heard about herbal supplements that have worked for someone we know. People swear by them: echinacea for a cold, ginkgo biloba for memory or the peppermint in the salve your aunt believes can ease chest congestion. Over the past decade, use of herbal supplements has jumped.

While many of those users may be skeptical, they figure, "Hey, these things are natural; what harm could they do?"

As it turns out, in some cases they can do a lot of harm, and a surprising number of people are putting themselves at risk by using herbal supplements without being informed about their actual benefits and potential dangers.

Though some herbs such as Ginkgo, Echinacea and Chamomile have been studied and seem to be mildly effective in treating certain symptoms or disorders, the same can't be said of all herbs. Herbs are better used as a complementary treatment, alongside traditional drugs, and under the guidance of a medical practitioner. Herbs alone might not be enough to help you fight a serious problem, but false advertisement and lack of regulations might trick you into thinking otherwise. This can be a dangerous assumption and might lead to serious problems.

Herbs might interact with prescription drugs in serious ways, but many people discount these effects. Many people don't inform their doctors about supplements they're taking and might risk their health in the process. Also, some interactions are well known, but it's difficult to say what happens with less-known herbs. Certain herbs can cancel the effects of prescription drugs. For example, St. John's Wort, a popular over-the-counter treatment for depression, can interfere with a large number of drugs — including certain blood thinners, cardiac drugs, antidepressants and HIV and cancer medications.

A patient might believe that taking a certain supplement will relieve pain, or boost immunity. In fact, it may conflict with a drug the doctor prescribed, or it may simply negate the benefit of the drug (or vice versa.) An example of this is the use of drugs for gastro-reflux disease (GERD), called proton pump inhibitors (like Prilosec, Nexium, Previcid, and others), combined with some forms of calcium supplements taken to strengthen bones and teeth. The drug cancels out the benefits of the calcium.

There's No "Alternative" to Medicine

To avoid such complications, ask your doctor before you decide to try an herbal supplement, and be sure to disclose any supplements you're taking even if you're not asked. That can be particularly important when you're being prescribed a new medication. The message here is not to avoid all herbal supplements. Increasingly, Western medicine is improving because of discoveries about these alternative treatments. However, it's important to remember that they are essentially drugs, and the best way to use them is to separate fact from fiction first.

As I stated earlier, I do have an extensive background and knowledge in the area of Herbal Medicine and Homeopathy, so I have a respectful knowledge of their benefits to health. So don't take my thoughts as a blanket condemnation.

Despite the criticism of herbal medicine among mainstream medical professionals, it is wise to remember that many common drugs we use today were derived from plant-based sources. Scientists originally derived aspirin from willow bark; herbalists prescribe white willow for headaches and pain control. Digitalis, a drug prescribed for certain heart conditions, comes from an extract of potentially toxic foxglove flowers. While it's true that herbal supplement manufacturers often make bold or outrageous claims, critics shouldn't be so quick to dismiss herbal medicine as quackery.

And, I would be remiss to add another key point:

Distrust in physicians often leads many people to place strong confidence in herbs and natural supplements. From my days behind the counter at my own "Herb Store", I saw all too often, how many people came there looking for a "therapeutic relationship" with someone who seemed to care about them. Not finding this caring relationship with many medical doctors, folks are willing to forgo care from their own doctor by refusing surgery or other treatment. In some cases, they will withdraw from care all together, or worse, not seeking it in the first place. Needless to say, this is a recipe for disaster.

Based on more years of experience that I care to admit, here are some of my "golden rules". Follow them and you'll never go wrong:

- ALWAYS keep in mind that qualified herbalists know when a condition is best seen by a doctor or another health professional.
- Avoid **anyone** who tells you it's not necessary to tell your medical doctor that you are taking herbs or natural supplements.
- If your medical doctor ever prescribes a drug for you, immediately make him/her aware of **all** herbs or supplements you are taking.
- If your doctor "doesn't believe in herbs", then that's not your doctor. Find a medical doctor who will respect your viewpoint, and support your efforts to use herbs or supplements responsibly.
- If you are around and I should have a medical "crisis", take me to the hospital, not the Herb Store!
- There is **no** "alternative" for the proper medical care of a serious medical condition. You should always be under the supervision of a medical doctor.
- There are not many well controlled research studies that have shown a positive effect for CAM approaches and people should be careful not to get sucked into things just because they think they make sense or for which there is little or no evidence of usefulness.

STRESS AND
YOUR HEALTH

THESE are the times that try men's souls.

—THOMAS PAINE – *The Crisis*
December 23, 1776

I f you are like most of us, you are probably really going through it, trying to survive and maintain during these turbulent times.

Economic turmoil (e.g., increased unemployment, foreclosures, loss of investments and other financial distress) can result in a whole host of negative health effects–both physical and mental. It can be particularly devastating to your emotional and mental well-being. Although each of us is affected differently by economic troubles, these problems can add tremendous stress, which in turn can substantially increase the risk for developing such problems.

Many people are aware of the alarming number of folks who are suffering with a wide range of what are now considered common health problems. High blood pressure; acid reflux; diabetes; ulcers; arthritis; obesity; asthma; and many others make up the list. It is a common belief that these are conditions expected at some point in life.

However, on closer examination, it seems that there is a mysterious culprit that is a factor in all of these problems: **STRESS.**

Stress isn't just a state of mind — it can affect your entire body. 75% to 90% of all doctor's office visits are said to be for stress-related ailments and complaints. Most physicians agree that stress can make many medical conditions worse or even trigger a relapse of a condition, stress, however, is usually not the root cause of a disease. Other factors such as genes, physical environment, etc. may cause the disease, but stress can make it worse.

Stress is the body's reaction to any change that requires an adjustment or response. The body reacts to these changes with physical, mental, and emotional responses.

Stress can trigger the body's response to perceived threat or danger, the Fight-or-Flight response. During this reaction, certain hormones like adrenalin and cortisol are released, speeding the heart rate, slowing digestion, shunting blood flow to major muscle groups, and changing various other autonomic nervous functions, giving the body a burst of energy and strength. Originally named for its ability to enable us to physically fight or run away when faced with danger, it's now activated in situations where neither response is appropriate, like in traffic or during a stressful day at work. When the perceived threat is gone, systems are designed to return to normal function via the relaxation response, but in our times of chronic stress, this often doesn't happen enough, causing damage to the body.

Stress and Your Health

Stress that continues without relief can lead to a condition called distress — a negative stress reaction. Distress can lead to physical symptoms including headaches, upset stomach, elevated blood pressure, chest pain, and problems sleeping. Research suggests that stress also can bring on or worsen certain symptoms or diseases.

To understand what stress does to us, imagine you lived tens of thousands of years ago, at a time when humans were threatened by hungry animals such as saber-toothed tigers and wolves. Our caveman ancestors had to be able to react instantly, either by fighting the beasts or running away.

So humans evolved the ability to respond to a stressful situation instantly, by preparing the body for "fight or flight." Under sudden stress, you will get a burst of exceptional strength and endurance, as your body pumps out stress **hormones**:

- Your heart speeds up
- Blood flow to your brain and muscles increases up to 400 percent
- Your digestion stops (so it doesn't use up energy that's needed elsewhere)
- Your muscle tension increases
- You breathe faster, to bring more oxygen to your muscles
- Sometimes we can still benefit from this "fight or flight" response–like the case of a mother whose child was pinned under a concrete slab during a tornado. Under stress, she found the strength to lift the huge slab with her bare hands, even though it later took three men to move it.

But much of the time in modern life, the "fight or flight" response won't help. Yet those stress hormones still flood your system, preparing you for physical action. And if you are under stress frequently, it can harm your physical health.

Cortisol is an important hormone in the body, secreted by the adrenal glands and involved in the following functions and more:

Proper glucose metabolism
- Regulation of blood pressure
- Insulin release for blood sugar maintenance
- Immune function
- Inflammatory response
- Normally, it's present in the body at higher levels in the morning, and at it's lowest at night. Although stress isn't the only reason that cortisol is secreted into the bloodstream, it has been termed "the stress hormone" because it's also secreted in higher levels during the body's 'fight or flight' response to stress, and is responsible for several stress-related changes in the body. Small increases of cortisol have some positive effects:

A quick burst of energy for survival reasons
- Heightened memory functions
- A burst of increased immunity
- Lower sensitivity to pain
- Helps maintain homeostasis in the body
- While cortisol is an important and helpful part of the body's response to stress, it's important that the body's relaxation re-

sponse to be activated so the body's functions can return to normal. Unfortunately, in our current high-stress culture, the body's stress response is activated so often that functioning often doesn't have a chance to return to normal, producing chronic stress.

One side effect of increased cortisol in the body can be weight gain, especially in the abdominal area, which can bring more negative health consequences than fat stored in other areas of the body.

Excess cortisol can be stimulated by physical stress such as over-exercising, lack of sleep, dieting, and poor nutrition, mental stress such as a high stress work environment, and emotional stress such as a death of a family member or even just too many demands on your time.

Stress is a natural part of life but its effects don't have to be a natural part of your health.

MENTAL ILLNESS

In any given year 26 percent of American adults suffer from mental disorders.

Think about it, when you walk down the street, at least one out of every four or five people you pass is suffering from some form of mental illness.

As Congresswoman Gifford continues to make a most surprising recovery, in a jail cell somewhere in Arizona awaiting what seems to be an almost certain fate, is a 22-year old young man, after shooting a total of 17 people and killing 6 of them.

Several of Jared Loughner's classmates and instructors at Pima Community College noticed his erratic behavior, had him removed from school, and notified his parents. Why was no one able to get him into treatment? A leading psychologist says our fear and misunderstanding of mental illness prevents us from stepping in before tragedies occur.

I believe that it is way past time for us to look at the state of mental health care in this country. Especially regarding emotional and mental illness, there are so many people who are unable to seek treatment because they may be unable to navigate the system in order to receive social services or they just don't have enough money to pay for treatment if they fall into middle class incomes because insurance rarely covers mental issues effectively. It must be remembered also that in the 1970's the doors to the mental hospitals were closed to the indigent and those people flooded the streets with nowhere to live, and no place to receive help. Not to mention that we, as a society turn a blind eye.

One of the greatest, and most undertreated, threats affecting Americans today is Mental Illness. Hundreds of millions of people worldwide are affected by mental, neurological or behavioral problems at any time.

In keeping with the prevalence of health disparities and inequities in practically every other area of health, the African American community suffers disproportionately from both mental health and mental health treatment.

One in four patients visiting a health service has at least one mental, neurological or behavioral disorder, but most of these disorders are neither diagnosed nor treated.

African Americans account for only 2% of psychiatrists, 2% of psychologists, and 4% of social workers in the United States.

Mental illnesses affect, and are affected by, chronic conditions such as cancer, heart and cardiovascular diseases, diabetes and HIV/AIDS. Untreated, they bring about unhealthy behavior, non-compliance with prescribed medical regimens, diminished immune functioning, and poor prognosis.

Compounding this disparity in mental health is the existence of a pervasive stigma that is held widely in the African American community: "they might think I'm crazy"!

Information is the Best Medicine

The stigma that engulfs African Americans on the issue of mental illness has its' origins deep in the annals of slave history in America.

One scientific report went so far as to deliberately falsify the black insanity rates from the 1840 U.S. census to show that the further North blacks lived, the higher their rates of lunacy strong evidence, of course, that freedom drove blacks crazy!

Over 150 years after the 1840 census, there are still important gaps and paradoxes in our knowledge of the mental health status of the African American population.

African Americans are disproportionately exposed to social conditions considered to be important risk factors for physical and mental illness.

African Americans frequently lack a usual source of health care as a focal point for treatment. For many African Americans, the emergency room is generally the source of primary care treatment. As a result, mental health care occurs frequently in emergency rooms and psychiatric hospitals. These settings and limited treatment available there, undermine the delivery of high-quality mental health care. I was just at one last week with a friend and his wife in support of their daughter.

Adaptive traditions have sustained African Americans through long periods of hardship imposed by the larger society. There is a historical tendency to "cope" and "adapt" through a myriad of mechanisms. Among them are food, smoking; illicit drugs; violence; and sex, just to name a few. For some, it is a total withdrawal from social interactions.

I always remember a childhood friend, who had an "Uncle John", who sat in the same chair, by the window, day in, day out, for as long as I can remember. I can still hear my friend's mother telling visitors to the house, "Oh, don't mind him, that's just Uncle John. He won't bother you, he harmless".

Less than half of African American adults with mental illness seek treatment for mental health problems, and less than one third of their children receive treatment.

The lack in receiving treatment is due in part to the stigma that surrounds mental disorders in the African American community.

African American communities across the United States are more culturally diverse now that any other time in history with increasing numbers of immigrants from African nations, the Caribbean, Central America and other countries. To ensure African American communities have access to adequate and affordable care, a better understanding of the complex role that cultural backgrounds and diverse experiences play in mental disorders in these communities is vital.

Because African Americans often turn to community – family, friends, neighbors, community groups and religious leaders – for help, the opportunity exists for community health services to collaborate with local churches and community groups to provide mental health care and education to families and individuals.

I think it is only fair and appropriate to recognize the efforts of Dr. Arthur Evans at the Philadelphia Department of Behavioral Health, who understands this, and is making tremendous strides in leading the nation in transforming how mental and behavioral health is delivered.

On the surface, the deep threat this issue poses to African American health may not be apparent. However, mental illnesses affect, and are affected by, chronic conditions such as cancer, heart and cardiovascular diseases, diabetes and HIV/AIDS. Untreated, they bring about unhealthy behavior, non-compliance with prescribed medical regimens, diminished immune functioning, and poor prognosis.

If this major public health issue is to be addressed effectively in the African American community, several things have to take place:

- More aggressive efforts in addressing Health Disparities and Inequities as a community
- Educate and involve Religious leaders in directing seekers of prayer to Mental Health Services
- Make mental health a part of dialogue in primary care settings
- Increase the availability of African American Mental Heath Providers
- Encourage compliance and continuation of treatment by family and friends
- Let elected official and policy makers know that we expect much more from them

CANCER 101

———————

Learning that you have cancer can come as a shock. How do you react? You may feel numb, frightened, or angry. You may not even believe what the doctor says. You may feel all alone, even if your friends and family are in the same room with you. These feelings are all normal.

For many people, the first few weeks after a cancer diagnosis are very hard. After you hear the word "cancer," you may have trouble breathing or listening to what is being said. When you are at home, you may have trouble thinking, eating, or sleeping.

If you're like most people, you're clueless about cancer.

Let's see if we can change that...

Cells are the building blocks of living things. Cancer grows out of normal cells in the body. Normal cells multiply when the body needs them, and die when the body doesn't need them. Cancer appears to occur when the growth of cells in the body are out of control and cells divide too quickly. It can also occur when cells "forget" how to die.

The body is made up of hundreds of millions of living cells. Normal body cells grow, divide, and die in an orderly fashion. During the early years of a person's life, normal cells divide faster to allow the person to grow. After the person becomes an adult, most cells divide only to replace worn-out or dying cells or to repair injuries.

Appropriate treatment for cancer depends on what kind of cancer you have. The type of cancer is determined by the organ the cancer starts in, the kind of cell from which it is derived, as well the appearance of the cancer cells. There are many different kinds of cancers. Cancer can develop in almost any organ or tissue, such as the lung, colon, breast, skin, bones, or nerve tissue.

There are over 100 different types of cancer, and the type of cell that is initially affected classifies each one. There are five broad groups that are used to classify cancer:

1. **Carcinomas** are characterized by cells that affect parts of the body such as lung, breast, and colon cancer.
2. **Sarcomas** are characterized by cells that are located in bone, cartilage, fat, connective tissue, muscle, and other supportive tissues.
3. **Lymphomas** are cancers that begin in the lymph nodes and immune system.
4. **Leukemias** are cancers that begin in the bone marrow and often accumulate in the bloodstream.
5. **Adenocarcinomas** are cancers that develop from adenomas; generally considered benign tumors that arise in the thyroid, the pituitary gland, the adrenal gland, and other glandular tissues.

Cancer 101

Cancer harms the body when damaged cells divide uncontrollably to form lumps or masses of tissue called tumors (except in the case of leukemia where cancer prohibits normal blood function by abnormal cell division in the blood stream). Tumors can grow and interfere with the digestive, nervous, and circulatory systems, and they can release hormones that alter body function. Tumors that stay in one spot and demonstrate limited growth are generally considered to be benign.

There are many causes of cancers, including:

- Benzene and other chemicals
- Certain poisonous mushrooms and a type of poison that can grow on peanut plants (aflatoxins)
- Certain viruses
- Radiation
- Sunlight
- Tobacco

However, the cause of many cancers remains unknown.

The most common cause of cancer-related death is lung cancer.

The three most common cancers in men in the United States are:

1. Prostate
2. Lung cancer
3. Colon cancer

In women in the U.S., the three most common cancers are:

1. Breast cancer
2. Colon cancer
3. Lung cancer

Some cancers are more common in certain parts of the world. For example, in Japan, there are many cases of gastric cancer, but in the U.S. this type of cancer is pretty rare. Differences in diet may play a role.

Some other types of cancers include:

- Brain cancer
- Cervical cancer
- Hodgkin's lymphoma
- Kidney cancer
- Leukemia
- Liver cancer
- Non-Hodgkin's lymphoma
- Ovarian cancer
- Skin cancer
- Testicular cancer
- Thyroid cancer
- Uterine cancer

Symptoms of cancer depend on the type and location of the tumor. For example, lung cancer can cause coughing, shortness of breath, or chest pain. Colon cancer often causes diarrhea, constipation, and blood in the stool.

Cancer 101

Some cancers may not have any symptoms at all. In certain cancers, such as gallbladder cancer, symptoms often do not start until the disease has reached an advanced stage.

The following symptoms can occur with most cancers:

- Chills
- Fatigue
- Fever
- Loss of appetite
- Malaise
- Night sweats
- Weight loss

Half of all men and one-third of all women in the US will develop cancer during their lifetimes.

Being diagnosed with cancer is a *process*. It doesn't happen all at once. If you have just gotten word you may have cancer, probably have cancer, or even do have cancer, the type and stage of your cancer may still be unknown. In many cases, the doctors can be pretty sure of the type and stage just from the initial studies, but sometimes even the type of cancer is in question for quite some time.

Cancer treatment depends on the type of cancer, the stage of the cancer (how much it has spread), age, health status, and additional personal characteristics. There is no single treatment for cancer, and patients often receive a combination of therapies and palliative care. Treatments usually fall into one of the following categories: surgery, radiation, chemotherapy, immunotherapy, or hormone therapy.

INFORMATION IS THE BEST MEDICINE

A few pointers:

1. **Until a pathologist has examined a sample of your tumor from surgery or a biopsy, the exact type of cancer may not be known.** For cancer in a number of organs, the vast majority of cancers are of the same type. For example almost all prostate cancers are adenocarcinomas and a large majority of cervical cancers are squamous cell carcinoma. The grade and other cellular factors influencing your prognosis will also not be known until a sample of your tumor is examined. In a quite a few cases this may not happen until after surgery to remove the primary tumor.

2. **Before surgery to remove the primary tumor, the staging is only presumptive.** The exact degree of spread is often impossible to determine until the pathologist examines the surgical specimen. The actual degree of lymph node involvement is often not known until after surgery. For some cancers, such as breast cancer, surgical procedures are done just to determine what stage your cancer is in, and/or whether the nodes are involved.

Despite these uncertainties, you can start researching the staging and treatment of the type of cancer you are suspected of having well before the final diagnosis is in. If you do, you will get far more out of your doctor visits, and you will be ready to make the important decisions ahead. Be prepared for surprises as new information comes in. Cancer is a real roller coaster, and you may have to change your direction many times before you are done.

Today, millions of people are living with cancer or have had cancer.

Cancer 101

The risk of developing most types of cancer can be reduced by changes in a person's lifestyle, for example, quitting smoking, limiting time in the sun, being physically active, and eating a better diet. The sooner a cancer is found and treated, the better the chances are for living for many years.

A LOOK AT
LIVER CANCER

The number of new cases of hepatocellular carcinoma (HCC), a type of primary liver cancer, has increased in the U.S. over the past several years, reaching an incidence rate of 3.2 cases per 100,000 persons in 2006, according to the latest figures reported by the Centers for Disease Control and Prevention (CDC) in the May 7, 2010 issue of *Morbidity and Mortality Weekly Report*. Blacks and people in the 50-59 year age group had the largest annual percentage increases in HCC.

In fact, I have lost a sister, and several other people close to me from liver cancer. Almost all of them did not understand how they might have avoided their situation.

The liver is the largest organ inside the body. It lies under your right ribs, just below the right lung. If you were to poke your fingers up under your right ribs, you would almost touch your liver.

The liver is shaped like a pyramid and is divided into right and left lobes. Unlike most other organs, the liver gets blood from two sources.

A Look at Liver Cancer

The hepatic artery supplies the liver with blood that is rich in oxygen. The portal vein carries nutrient-rich blood from the intestines to the liver.

You cannot live without your liver. It has many vital jobs:

- It breaks down and stores many of the nutrients absorbed from the intestine.
- It makes some of the clotting factors needed to stop bleeding from a cut or injury.
- It makes bile that goes into the intestine to help absorb nutrients.
- It plays an important part in getting rid of toxic wastes from the body.

The liver has many other functions. Some of the functions are: to produce substances that break down fats, convert glucose to glycogen, produce urea (the main substance of urine), and make certain amino acids (the building blocks of proteins), filter harmful substances from the blood (such as alcohol), storage of vitamins and minerals (vitamins A, D, K and B12) and maintain a proper level or glucose in the blood. The liver is also responsible for producing cholesterol. It produces about 80% of the cholesterol in your body. Although these are all important jobs that the liver performs they are but a few. Remember there are more than 500 functions!

Because the liver is made up of different types of cells, many types of tumors can form in the liver. Some of these are cancer and some are not. Tumors that are cancer are called *malignant*. The medical word for tumors that are not cancer is *benign*. These tumors have different causes and are treated different ways. The outlook for your health or your recovery (*prognosis*) depends on what type of tumor you have.

Liver cancer is the third most common cancer in the world. A deadly cancer, liver cancer will kill almost all patients who have it within a year. In 2000, it was estimated that there were about 564,000 new cases of liver cancer worldwide, and a similar number of patients died as a result of this disease. About three-quarters of the cases of liver cancer are found in Southeast Asia (China, Hong Kong, Taiwan, Korea, and Japan).

Hepatocellular carcinoma (HCC): This is the most common form of liver cancer in adults. It begins in the *hepatocytes*, the main type of liver cell. About 3 out of 4 cancers that start in the liver are this type. HCC can have different growth patterns.

Bile duct cancers (cholangiocarcinomas): Bile duct cancers account for 1 or 2 out of every 10 cases of liver cancer. These cancers start in the small tubes (called bile ducts) that carry bile to the gallbladder.

Cancers that begin in blood vessels in the liver (angiosarcomas and hemangiosarcomas): These are rare cancers that start in the blood vessels of the liver. These tumors grow quickly. Often by the time they are found they are too widespread to be removed. Treatment may help slow the disease, but most patients do not live more than a year after these cancers are found.

Hepatoblastoma: This is a very rare kind of liver cancer that is usually found in children younger than 4 years old. About 70% of children with this disease have good outcomes with surgery and chemotherapy. The survival rate is greater than 90% for early-stage disease.

World wide the vast majority of primary liver cancer can be prevented by early (neonatal or childhood) immunization against infection with Hepatitis B virus. Hepatitis B vaccine has already prevented up to 30 million deaths from hepatoma or chronic liver disease and is probably one of the safest vaccines ever developed.

Most of the time when cancer is found in the liver it did not start there, but started somewhere else and spread to the liver. This is called *metastatic cancer*. This can happen to people with advanced breast cancer, colorectal cancer, lung cancer, and many other cancers, too. Under a microscope, theses cancer cells in the liver look like the cancer cells that they came from. If someone has lung cancer that has spread to the liver, the cancer cells in the liver will look and act like lung cancer cells and they will be treated the same way.

Most people don't have signs and symptoms in the early stages of primary liver cancer. When symptoms do appear, they may include:

- Losing weight without trying
- Loss of appetite
- Upper abdominal pain
- Nausea and vomiting
- General weakness and fatigue
- An enlarged liver
- Abdominal swelling
- Yellow discoloration of your skin and the whites of your eyes (jaundice)

The liver has a considerable reserve so that a very large part of it has to be diagnosed as non-functioning before it affects the whole body. Patients with liver failure often complain of swollen ankles or an increase in their abdominal girth, which is due to fluid leaking out of the blood vessels and accumulating in other tissue and body compartments.

Maintaining a steady glucose level also becomes increasingly difficult resulting in low blood sugar levels. This leaves a person feeling tired and unable to function well. Detoxification of ingested material is impacted leaving the brain at the mercy of unprocessed or poorly processed drugs and toxins. This results in "brain fog" which leaves a person unable to think clearly.

A classic feature of liver failure is jaundice: the yellow pigmentation of skin and the whites of our eyes (sclera) that results from deposition of bilirubin into these areas.

Bleeding and bruising is another common feature of liver failure. The body's blood vessels and other body tissues constantly sustain minor tears even without any antecedent trauma. The liver produces clotting factors, which are key to maintaining the integrity of the blood vessels and tissues.

It's important to meet your nutrition needs before, during, and after cancer treatment. You need the right amount of calories, protein, vitamins, and minerals. Getting the right nutrition can help you feel better and have more energy. However, you may be uncomfortable or tired, and you may not feel like eating.

You also may have side effects of treatment such as poor appetite, nausea, vomiting, or diarrhea. Your doctor, a registered dietitian, or another health care provider can advise you about ways to have a healthy diet.

Vitamin and mineral supplements may also help provide nutrients that your diet may not contain. Vitamins and minerals also offer a boost where the liver cancer may have depleted your body. In many situations, dietary supplements help support your immune system and reduce toxic side effects. Your dietitian may recommend daily dosages of various nutrients, including:

- Beta carotene
- Selenium
- Vitamin C
- Eicosapentaenoic acid (EPA)
- Vitamin E
- Others as appropriate

A LOOK AT
PROSTATE CANCER

<hr>

More than any other condition, Prostate Cancer comes up when it comes to the subject of Men's Health. And the PSA test is most commonly mentioned when it comes to prevention of Prostate Cancer.

The PSA test measures blood levels of a protein made by the prostate. Levels of less than 4.0 (nanograms of protein per milliliter of blood) are usually considered within the normal range, while levels of greater than 4.0 are said to show an increased risk for prostate cancer.

The prostate-specific antigen (PSA) screening test for early prostate cancer has been surrounded by controversy ever since it was introduced. To the surprise of many, there is no proof that the use of this blood test to screen symptom-free men will spare anyone a prostate cancer death. In short, cancer researchers do not know whether PSA screening saves more lives than it ruins.

First of all, let me be clear: **I'm not against prostate cancer screening.**

A Look at Prostate Cancer

I'm a tremendous supporter of the real American Cancer Society (ACS) recommendation, which is: Within the physician-patient relationship, men should be offered PSA screening and should be informed of the potential risks, as well as the potential benefits and be allowed to make a choice.

The prostate cancer outcomes from a huge study conducted by the National Cancer Institute, shows that close to 40% of men who undergo a radical prostatectomy (surgical removal of the prostate) will have a PSA relapse within two years.

If you have a group of men diagnosed as a result of PSA screening, 30-40% don't need to know that they have prostate cancer because it's meaningless in terms of risk to their health. And for somewhere between 30% and 40% of the men with prostate cancer, no matter what [treatment is given], the disease is not curable. And then maybe there are about 20% who actually benefit. These facts are from clinical studies done by credible researchers from credible institutions.

Men who are screened for prostate cancer are usually relieved when their prostate specific antigen [PSA] levels come back normal. But according to a new study in The New England Journal of Medicine, the results may be misleading. The study found that 15 percent of the men who had "normal" PSA levels still had prostate cancer. High-grade cancer was found in about 2.3 percent of those so-called "normal" men. It appears that the lower the PSA level, the smaller the risk—the likelihood of having cancer rises as PSA levels rise. But there is no clear PSA level at which a person can be guaranteed to be cancer-free. Some incidence of high-grade cancer—the most aggressive—was found at every PSA level.

At this point in time, it is not known for sure that having PSA screening actually reduces a man's risk of dying from prostate cancer.

So how do doctors differentiate between more and less aggressive versions of prostate cancer? By the way it feels. If your doctor can feel the cancer outside the prostate, that's a bad sign. But most prostate cancers detected today in men who are being screened are confined to the prostate. In those men, the main way they can tell something about the aggressiveness of the cancer is the by Gleason score, or the grade: the appearance of the cancer under the microscope. That can run from a number of 2 to a number of 10—10 being the most aggressive, 2 being the least.

In the United States this year, 1.4 million men will learn they have prostate cancer. So here's a guide for where to go in the days and weeks following a cancer diagnosis:

1. Get basic information about your cancer

Take notes and ask the questions that will help you understand enough to make good decisions.

2. Pick a doctor (Oncologist and/or Urologist)

Get referrals from friends who have had a similar experience and ask your primary doctor, who would they choose if it was for their son or father.

One of the first things your doctor will do is grade and stage the tumor. These ratings give an indication for how severe and fast growing the cancer is.

3. Learn how to read your lab reports.

Pathology reports have all sorts of valuable information, including how large the tumor is and whether it's spread. You don't have to be a doctor to learn how to read them.

4. Find alternative medicine for cancer

Many cancer patients want to know about herbs, supplements and other alternative approaches to fighting cancer, but doctors didn't learn much about those in medical school.

5. Find support groups

There are countless support groups for cancer patients.

6. Find out about clinical trials

At some point in your cancer treatment, you may decide to join a study of a new therapy. Some prostate cancers can grow and spread quickly, but most of the time, prostate cancer grows slowly. Autopsy studies show that many older men (and even younger men) who died of other diseases also had prostate cancer that never caused a problem during their lives. These studies showed that as many as 7 to 9 out of 10 men had prostate cancer by age 80. But neither they nor their doctors even knew they had it.

And now a word or two about a few some of the more popular "natural" remedies for prostate cancer:

Lycopene is a prominent member of the carotenoid family of chemical compounds, found in certain plants (like tomatoes. Research indicates that Lycopene's powerful antioxidant properties may also protect humans against certain disorders, such as prostate cancer and perhaps some forms of cancers, and coronary heart disease. In a recent trial, men with prostate cancer were randomly given Lycopene or a placebo for three weeks before undergoing prostate surgery. Upon examining the prostate tissue of these men it was found that those who received Lycopene had significantly less aggressive growth of cancer cells.

The high lignan content of **Flax Seed** is believed to be the defense mechanism against cancers that are primarily hormone-dependent. Lignans are a type of natural plant chemical (scientifically known as a phytochemical) contained within flaxseed. Lignans are considered to act as plant hormones. Researchers believe these plant hormones mimic the body's own estrogen type of cells and can block the formation of hormone-based tumors or growths. Flax seed has anywhere from 75-800 times more lignans than vegetables or other grain products.

Even though prostate cancer diagnosis alone is far from being a "death sentence", there are some things that you can do to reduce your risk. For example, reduction of caloric, intake increases in number of vegetables one eats—the same things that reduce risk of heart disease, stroke, and hypertension.

FINDING OUT YOU HAVE PROSTATE CANCER

W̶hen you hear the devastating news that you have cancer of the prostate, a small gland the size of a plum found in men below the bladder, it can be difficult to decide which of many treatment options are right for you. But the choice is vital: The prostate is responsible for making 10–30 percent of a man's semen and is involved in sexual performance and urination. When it malfunctions, it can cause a variety of health problems, from infection to severe back pain. The worst is prostate cancer. Dealing with "prostate" is often the first significant experience many black men have with the medical system. No wonder our decisions on how to handle it are often grounded in fear or mistrust and tend to be made with little or no information.

A 2003 study by researchers at Oxford University shows that a man diagnosed with cancer is unlikely to research his options and more likely to do as radio host and motivational speaker Les Brown admits he did: unquestioningly follow his doctor's advice—because, as Brown says, the patient mistakenly thinks the "doctor knows best." Each treatment—from hormone therapy to radiation to surgery/outright removal—has a different set of benefits and risks. Yet because men panic and do what the diagnosing doctor says, many will think of questions to ask only after they've already undergone a treatment and are dealing with its side effects. By then it is usually too late to pursue a different strategy.

Men also act out of another fear: impotence. They may do whatever the doctor says because they fear that if they don't, the condition will keep them from getting an erection. But prostate disease doesn't cause impotence—the treatments do. They can damage the veins or nerve pathways to the penis, making it difficult or impossible for a man to get it up.

After their initial diagnosis, most men actually have plenty of time to consider treatment options. Unlike many other cancers, prostate cancer generally progresses relatively slowly. Michael Barry, MD, chief of general medicine at Massachusetts General Hospital, found in 2004 that more men die with prostate cancer than of it because some tumors are small and grow very slowly, never endangering the man's life. Grace Lu-Yao, PhD, of Robert Wood Johnson Medical School, conducted a study that found that the great majority of prostate patients are going to die of something else, and that a large number do well with no initial treatment and indeed with no treatment long term.

In fact, according to the National Cancer Institute, almost every man diagnosed with lung cancer dies of it, but only 226 out of every 100,000 men over the age of 65 with prostate cancer die of prostate cancer. While options will vary according to your circumstances, you should follow this three-step approach to obtaining appropriate treatment as soon as your screening test comes back positive.

Step 1. Assess the Situation The process of being diagnosed with prostate cancer differs for every man. So when any screening test comes back positive, ask lots of questions. Among the most important: What additional tests or procedures do I need to determine definitively whether I have cancer? You may need as many as three tests, generally in this order: a digital rectal exam (DRE), a prostate-specific antigen (PSA) blood test and a biopsy, where a sample of tissue is removed and examined. Usually these are performed by your primary-care physician or a urologist, who specializes in problems of the urinary and reproductive systems. Sometimes test results are inconclusive and need repeating. Always take a family member or friend when you get the results of a biopsy—the information can be overwhelming. That person should be willing to be your ongoing "treatment partner," able to act as your second set of eyes and ears, ask questions, review information with you and accompany you on subsequent doctor visits. Any time you must attend an appointment alone, always take a notebook or tape recorder. A biopsy that's positive for cancer returns "scored" and "staged," assessments of the seriousness of the condition. The cancer "score," on what is known as the Gleason Scale, reflects how likely it will grow quickly and spread: 2–4 mildly aggressive; 5–7 moderately aggressive; 8–10 very aggressive.

The cancer is assigned to one of four "stages" based on how much is present and how far it has spread:

- **Stage I:** Early cancer that is too small to feel when the doctor examines your prostate.
- **Stage II:** The doctor can feel the tumor, but it is contained inside your prostate gland.
- **Stage III:** The cancer has spread to nearby tissues.
- **Stage IV:** The cancer has spread to the lymph nodes, bones, lungs or other areas in the body.

Step 2: Get a Second Opinion Ask your primary physician, urologist or cancer specialist (in the event you're sent to one immediately) how long you have to make your decisions. Getting a second opinion from another doctor is critical for obtaining the best care. Don't worry about upsetting your initial doctor: Second opinions are a crucial and expected part of the medical process. Doctors can interpret data differently, tend to be most knowledgeable about the treatments they've been trained to perform, and may even appreciate the perspective additional opinions bring. If you have been told your diagnosis is serious, time may be an issue and you may need to make a quicker decision. Seeking a second opinion after a prostate cancer diagnosis can sometimes mean the difference between radical surgery and what is called "watchful waiting": aggressively monitoring your condition before you settle on a treatment option. In some cases, doctors disagree on whether cancer is even present. If this happens, have doctors explain how he or she reached their conclusions. Also ask them to confer with each other to see if they can agree on one approach. If you are worried that the doctors might be cronies, schedule a consultation with a medical oncologist, a cancer treatment specialist who does not perform radiation or surgery but can oversee the treatment given by other specialists.

Step 3: Pick a Treatment Strategy Prostate cancer treatment is not "one size fits all." You should choose the best treatment for you with the help of your family and one or more doctors. These may include: a urologist; a medical oncologist, a cancer specialist who administers chemotherapy and hormone therapy, and who may coordinate treatment given by other doctors; a surgical oncologist, who performs surgeries to remove cancerous growths or tumors; and a radiation oncologist, who treats cancer with radiation. The doctors should always consider the grade and stage of your cancer, your age and general health, and your values and feelings about the potential benefits and harm of each option. Here are your alternatives, from most to least invasive. For more treatment-decision tools, contact the American Cancer Society (cancer.org or 800.ACS.1234).

SURGERY The surgical removal of the entire prostate gland is called a radical prostatectomy, where an incision is made either below the navel or below your rectum. Evidence shows that men who opt for this surgery may have a better chance for long-term survival than those who choose other options. Since surgery has the longest track record for keeping men cancer-free, it remains the treatment of choice of most men. Of course, the more of the cancer doctors can get out of your body, the greater your chances are of survival. Success also depends on the age of the patient and factors like whether he received hormone therapy prior to surgery or additional therapies such as radiation therapy either prior to or after the surgery. Unfortunately, because surgery can damage nerves involved in erection, it also has the greatest risk of impotence and problems with bowel function. After surgery, it can take two years or longer to recover, although some men recover sooner. Two newer surgical methods offer greater precision to minimize nerve damage: Laparoscopic surgery allows the surgeon to make several tiny incisions, the size of keyholes, to remove the prostate. Robotic procedures let surgeons operate with the help of mechanical "arms" while they watch on a video screen.

ADVANTAGES TO SURGICAL OPTIONS:

- All cancer cells growing in the prostate are removed.
- If the cancer hasn't spread beyond your prostate, you have a 90 percent chance of living at least 10 years afterward.

DISADVANTAGES:

- As with any major surgery, there is a chance of complications such as infection, pneumonia, blood clots and other problems, as well as the possibility of death.
- Impotence due to nerve damage is common.
- You may have stress incontinence, which means you can't hold your urine flow when there's increased bladder pressure—when you sneeze, cough, laugh or lift, or even simply when standing or walking.
- Even without a prostate, cancer can appear in other parts of your body. It is impossible to know if any of the cancer cells spread outside of the prostate before it was removed.

RADIATION Radiation therapy uses high doses of radiation to treat cancer. It is most effective when prostate cancer has not spread beyond the prostate gland or has spread only to nearby tissues, or as an option to help shrink the tumor or to reduce symptoms when a cure is not possible. Radiation is also used for men who cannot have surgery because of their age, health or personal choice. Five to eight years after treatment, survival rates for radiation therapy are equal to those of surgery when treatment is for cancer that has not spread beyond the prostate. There are two types of radiation therapy: External beam radiation: The radiation is focused on the prostate gland from outside the body—like getting an X-ray, but for a longer time. Treatments are generally given five days a week for about six to eight weeks on an outpatient basis. Each treatment appointment takes about 15 minutes, with most of this time for preparation. Seed implants: This treatment, called brachytherapy, involves placing radioactive seeds or pellets (about the size of a grain of rice) in or near the prostate tumor and leaving them there permanently. After several weeks or months, the radioactivity level of the implants eventually diminishes to nothing. The seeds then remain in the prostate, with no lasting effect.

ADVANTAGES:

- Major surgery can often be avoided.
- Rates of sexual problems such as erectile dysfunction (ED) and urinary problems are very low.
- No hospital stay
- No anesthesia risk

DISADVANTAGES:

- Impotence may develop up to two years later in some patients and can be a permanent side effect.
- If the prostate cancer doesn't respond, the cancer cannot be retreated with radiation.
- Bowel function may not return to normal after treatment is complete.
- Since nerves that help a man have an erection are right next to the prostate, radiation may damage them.

CRYOTHERAPY The newest treatment for prostate cancer is cryotherapy. This strategy involves freezing and then thawing the tissues of the prostate gland, dehydrating and destroying the cells using a minimally invasive surgical procedure. Almost 98 percent of patients who are treated with cryotherapy are cancer-free after one year, and 95 percent are still alive at the five-year mark.

ADVANTAGES:

- Freezing triggers antibodies that destroy cancer cells.
- Effective when radiation fails
- Can be used if you are not healthy enough for surgery
- Little loss of blood from procedure

DISADVANTAGES:

- New treatment, so not a lot is known about long-term effectiveness
- Few urologists are trained to perform it.

- Not effective in late-stage prostate cancer
- Temporary impotence

CHEMOTHERAPY Chemotherapy is a drug treatment that is used to try to kill cancer cells or to stop them from spreading. This treatment is an option for men whose prostate cancer has spread (metastasized) to other parts of the body, or for those who have used hormone therapy (see below) to slow the growth of their cancer. Chemotherapy drugs are usually injected into the blood, after which they travel around the body, attacking cancer cells wherever they find them.

ADVANTAGES:

- Reduces the odds of your cancer returning if taken after another treatment for prostate cancer, such as surgery or hormone therapy(see below)
- Slows the spread of cancer
- Can be used in combination with hormone therapy
- Relieves pain if cancer has spread to bones

DISADVANTAGES:

- Weakens immune system and increases chance of infections
- Often causes nausea and vomiting
- Weight loss frequently occurs.
- Tingling and loss of sensation in hands and feet

HORMONE THERAPY Hormone therapy starves cancer cells by slowing or stopping the production of the male hormone testosterone, which is vital to the growth and function of a normal prostate, but which automatically feeds cancer cells because it cannot distinguish between them and healthy cells. A series of injections is given every three, four, six or 12 months. While hormone therapy causes prostate cancer to shrink in 85 to 90 percent of advanced prostate cancer patients, it does not cure the disease. In addition, the effects last only between 24 and 36 months.

ADVANTAGES:

- Causes tumors to shrink
- Slows the growth of cancer
- Lowers PSA count

DISADVANTAGES:

- Decreased sex drive
- Swelling or tenderness of the chest tissue
- Constipation or diarrhea No or decreased appetite

CLINICAL TRIAL A clinical trial is a research study where you are given drugs or treatments not yet approved by the FDA for prostate cancer. These treatments are experimental and sometimes may involve you getting a placebo (sugar pill) and not the actual drug, so before signing up it is important to ask if you are receiving treatment or just being observed. Many clinical trials divide the patients in two groups, with one receiving the actual drug or treatment and the other receiving a sugar pill, in order to compare the results.

ADVANTAGES:

- Access to leading doctors in the field of prostate cancer research
- Possible benefit from drugs or treatments that are not available to other patients

DISADVANTAGES:

- You may receive a treatment that has no benefit.
- Since your treatment is unapproved, you may experience unknown side effects.

COMPLEMENTARY AND ALTERNATIVE MEDICINE (CAM) Many people are turning to natural herbs and supplements to treat their health problems, including prostate cancer. While ongoing National Institutes of Health research suggests that specific nutrients, such as Vitamin E, may ward off cancer, no CAM treatment has yet been proven to treat or cure prostate cancer. What's more, it's not always easy to tell which products may be unsafe, interact negatively with other medications or affect your overall cancer, so it's best to talk with your doctor or naturopath before taking any dietary or herbal product. Keep in mind that supplements and herbs are not approved by the FDA for treatment of cancer.

ADVANTAGES:

- May help alleviate the side effects of cancer treatments, such as nausea, pain and fatigue

DISADVANTAGES:

- They may interfere with how well other medicines you are taking work in your body.

WATCHFUL WAITING Many prostate cancers are small and grow slowly. If this is your diagnosis, it may not be necessary to treat your prostate cancer. In watchful waiting, you obtain no treatment, but you should see your doctor every three to six months for a PSA and digital rectal exam. If there continues to be no sign that the cancer is growing, you may continue to forgo treatment. The best candidates for watchful waiting are older men whose tumors are small and slow-growing, as indicated by low scoring and low stage, since most men with prostate cancer die of something else.

ADVANTAGES:

- No recovery issues or complications found in other treatments

DISADVANTAGES:

- Prostate cancer can grow and spread outside the prostate before your next doctor's visit.

WILL YOU STILL BE ABLE TO GET IT UP?

The risks of impotence vary according to the procedure; surgery and radiation pose the greatest threat. If you choose surgery, studies show that rates of impotence range from less than 15 percent to more than 80 percent, depending on your age and the experience of the surgeon. While radiation causes less impotence, surgery has better survival rates beyond 10 years. Hormone therapy won't cause impotence, but it may change your sexual desire by eliminating testosterone, a hormone that controls male sex drive. Most times this can be treated with medication for erectile dysfunction.

Chemotherapy might affect your ability to get and keep an erection, but this is usually temporary. You'll usually regain your sexual function within a few weeks of ending treatment. Success rates of such erectile dysfunction drugs as Viagra are higher in younger prostate patients and work better if you do not have a history of cigarette smoking, hypertension, high cholesterol and coronary artery disease.

Also, don't be surprised if you and your doctor have a different idea of what counts as an erection. As you make your way back to full sexual strength, talk to your urologist about your options for penile rehabilitation therapy. This involves an implant or a pump to help achieve an erection and is used in men who don't respond to oral medication for impotence.

ABOUT PROSTATE SCREENINGS FOR CANCER

For such a small gland (it's roughly the size of a walnut), the prostate has a very important job. If a man didn't have a prostate, the sperm couldn't survive. The main purpose of the prostate is to produce fluid and other compounds that help support sperm survival.

Prostate cancer affects many men each year. Screening includes a digital rectal exam, tests for prostate-specific antigen (PSA), and transrectal ultrasonography (TRUS). Each of these tests takes less than half an hour to perform.

The age-old question is, "Are they effective"?

New Mayo Clinic research studied the association between prostate-specific antigen (PSA) levels and prostate size and found that routine annual evaluation of prostate growth is not necessarily a predictor for the development of prostate cancer. However the study suggests that if a man's PSA level is rising quickly, a prostate biopsy is reasonable to determine if he has prostate cancer. Researchers are working on developing effective methods to screen for prostate cancer. However, it has not yet been shown that screening for prostate cancer decreases the chances of dying from prostate cancer.

Prostate cancer is the most common type of cancer found in American men, other than skin cancer. The American Cancer Society estimates that there will be about 179,300 new cases of prostate cancer in the United States this year, and about 37,000 men will die of this disease. For an American man, the lifetime risk of dying from prostate cancer is 3.4%.

Although men of any age can get prostate cancer, it is found most often in men over age 50. In fact, more than 8 of 10 men with prostate cancer are over the age of 65.

African-American men are at higher risk than Caucasian men. Men with a family history of prostate cancer are at higher risk too. Family history means that your father or a brother had prostate cancer.

The prostate gland is part of the male reproductive system. The prostate makes a fluid that mixes with sperm and other fluids during ejaculation. A normal prostate is about the size of a walnut.

Your doctor may examine your prostate by putting a gloved, lubricated finger a few inches into your rectum to feel your prostate gland. This is called a digital rectal exam. A normal prostate feels firm. If there are hard spots on the prostate, your doctor may suspect cancer. A more sensitive test measures prostate-specific antigen, or PSA, a protein manufactured by the prostate gland. An elevated level indicates an abnormality of the prostate.

An elevated PSA can be due to benign prostatic hypertrophy (an enlarged prostate), which affects nearly all men as they grow old. It can also signal prostatitis, an inflammation of the prostate. Both conditions may or may not warrant treatment, depending on the severity of symptoms. Neither problem is potentially fatal. But a high PSA level could indicate cancer.

An abnormal PSA test often leads to a biopsy to determine if cancer is present. In recent years, health professionals have questioned whether the PSA test is an effective way of detecting prostate cancer. Does it miss too many cancers? Does it lead to too many unnecessary biopsies? Is there a better way to screen for prostate cancer?

Although the PSA test is not perfect, it is the best currently available test for early detection of prostate cancer. Prostate Specific Antigen (PSA) is a protein made in the prostate. Normally, very little should be found in the blood. Rising levels of PSA in the blood indicate a problem with the prostate, which could be cancer but could also be an enlarged prostate (BPH).

While the PSA test is considered a major advance in diagnosing early-stage prostate cancer, it has some drawbacks. For 100 men over 50 at average risk for prostate cancer, the following would be found if they all had a PSA test:

Ten of the 100 men would have a PSA level higher than normal (over 4.0). The 10 men would need further testing to clarify their abnormal levels.

- Three of the 10 men would be found to have prostate cancer.
- Seven of the 10 men would be found not to have prostate cancer. They would have an elevated PSA for other reasons—most likely an enlarged prostate (BPH).

About Prostate Screenings for Cancer

- Ninety of the 100 men would have PSA levels in the normal range (less than 4.0).
- One or 2 of these 90 men would be found to have significant prostate cancer that becomes life threatening.
- This shows that the PSA test is moderately sensitive. Of 100 men with prostate cancer, it will detect only about 70 of them. But the positive predictive value of the PSA test is low. Only 3 out of 10 positive results were cancer. And 7 out of 10 positive PSA results (i.e., greater than 4.0) are false-positive results; this means that 2 out of 3 men who are told that they may have cancer after taking the PSA test actually do not have it. When the PSA is greater than 10.0, the test is more accurate. There is about a 50-50 chance of having cancer at this level of PSA!

Other things you and your doctor may want to consider:

- **Your age.** Doctors may use Age-adjusted PSA ranges to account for the natural increase in PSA with age when considering further testing.
- **The size of your prostate.** PSA Density is a measure that relates your PSA level to the size of your prostate, to account for the increase in PSA caused by prostate enlargement.
- **Your weight.** Body Mass Index, a measure of obesity, may also be a factor. The relationship between obesity and lower PSA levels may cause doctors to miss early prostate cancer cases in overweight men.
- **Ejaculation** within 48 hours before taking a PSA test can also cause a higher reading of your PSA level.

Refinements of the PSA test have been developed to reduce the number of false positive results. If your PSA is found to be high, ask your primary healthcare practitioner to discuss your cancer risk and the possible use of other evaluations of PSA before having a biopsy. Men should be counseled about the benefits and risks of detecting and treating an indolent tumor (this cancer may not have caused symptoms). The treatment may cause urinary and sexual problems.

Keep in mind that the ultimate goal of the PSA test is *not* to decide who should be biopsied and who should not. It is to save lives.

BREAST CANCER AND
THE ENVIRONMENT

===========

Many of the established risk factors for breast cancer—such as earlier menstrual cycle, later menopause, childlessness, and delayed childbearing—are ones women cannot change. And established risk factors do not account for all breast cancer cases. We simply do not know as much as we should about one of the overlooked factors.

Although the American Cancer Society estimates that environmental pollution causes 6% of all cancer deaths — or about 34,000 lost lives each year — they don't offer specific advice on which chemicals to avoid to reduce breast cancer risk.

Many people are now looking at our increasingly polluted environment as a possible culprit. Breast cancer incidence in the United States has risen since World War II, when industry began pumping out pesticides, plastics, solvents, and other chemicals, leaving residues in our air, water, and soil. Laboratory studies suggest that many of these chemicals may cause breast tumors, hasten their growth, or leave mammary glands more vulnerable to carcinogens.

A woman's lifetime risk of breast cancer is 1 in 8—representing a dramatic increase since the 1930s, when the first reliable cancer incidence data were established. Between 1973 and 1998 alone, breast cancer incidence rates in the United States increased by more than 40 percent. Strikingly, the increasing incidence of breast cancer since the 1930s parallels the proliferation of synthetic chemicals. Today, approximately 85,000 synthetic chemicals are registered for use in the United States, more than 90 percent of which have never been tested for their effects on human health.

The United States has seen a decline in breast cancer incidence in 2003 and 2004; a change that has been largely attributed to post-menopausal women discontinuing their hormone replacement therapy after research showed that it can cause breast cancer.

A report by the Breast Cancer Fund presents a comprehensive summary of the scientific data on the environmental causes of breast cancer. The report catalogues the growing evidence linking breast cancer to, among other factors, synthetic hormones in pharmaceuticals, cosmetics and meat; pesticides in food; solvents in household cleaning products; BPA in food containers; flame retardants in furniture; and radiation from medical treatments. The report also highlights impacts on the most vulnerable populations (including infants, pregnant women, African-American women and factory workers).

A number of studies suggest that such claims are not unfounded. Nationally, a 1987 study by the United Church of Christ's Commission on Racial Justice found Blacks were four times were more likely to live in areas with toxic and hazardous waste sites than Whites. A 1992 investigation by the *National Law Journal* found that when government does enforce environmental regulation and fine companies, fines are much higher in White communities than in Black ones. In Louisiana, reports by the US Commission on Civil Rights and an unreleased report by the US Environmental Protection Agency (EPA) Region Six, have raised concerns about the location of chemical plants and their possible impact on the health of their neighbors, who are primarily people of color.

These reports, and a host of activities by environmental justice groups nationwide, prompted President Clinton in 1993 to sign an executive order directing federal agencies to examine policies for disproportionate impact on people of color. As part of these efforts, the Clinton Administration set up the Office of Environmental Justice at the EPA.

Here are 9 Breast Cancer **environmental prevention** tips, which I came across:

1. **Avoid**: Toxic cosmetics, skin care products and sunscreens.

   Why: Unfortunately, these products contain carcinogens, hormone disruptors and a long list of other ingredients that may be linked to certain cancers.

   Choose: Healthy sunscreens and skin care cosmetics.

2. **Avoid**: All Teflon and non-stick coated cook and bakeware.

   Why: At 680°F Teflon pans release at least six toxic gases, including two carcinogens, two global pollutants, and MFA, a chemical lethal to humans at low doses.

Choose: Cook with cast iron cookware or high-quality stainless steel.

3. **Avoid:** Smoking, second hand smoke and car exhaust (avoid Polycyclic Aromatic Hydrocarbon, also known as PAH's)

   Why: The chemicals in cigarettes and cigarette smoke contain poisons, carcinogens and heavy, toxic metals.

   Choose: Clean air

4. **Avoid**: Toxic dry cleaning containing PERC (Perchloroethylene)

   Why: The EPA identifies PERC as a known human toxin. It usually enters the body through inhalation and remains stored in fat tissue, impairs neurological function, along with a higher cancer risk.

   Choose: Green dry cleaners.

5. **Avoid:** BPA exposure (bisphenol A) in plastics.

   Why: Pre-natal exposure to BPA may be linked to adult hormonal cancers, like breast and prostate cancers.

   Choose: Glass baby bottles, as well as BPA-free water bottles and BPA free canned food.

6. **Avoid:** Being still, sedentary, couch potato.

Choose: Exercise daily – whether it's walking, running, yoga, ...you decide.

Why: Reduces the risk of breast cancer by lowering estradiol and progesterone, two ovarian hormones linked to breast cancer tumor production.

7. **Avoid:** Toxic water.

    Why: Most water contains arsenic, fluoride, chlorine and other unhealthy toxins.

    Choose: Filtered drinking water.

8. **Avoid:** Toxic pesticides and weed killers:

    Why: Commonly used lawn care products contain endocrine disruptors and carcinogens, which have been implicated in increased risk for breast cancer as well as other health problems.

    Choose: Natural pesticides, that contain no endocrine disruptors or carcinogens.

9. **Avoid:** Toxic Food

    Why: Food is over processed with additives, preservatives, poisonous pesticides and fungicides and heavy metals, resulting in very little nutritional value. People are eating products instead of whole food.

    Choose: Organic whole food.

The poor are most likely to be exposed not only to the worst quality, the most noise, the worst water, and to hazardous wastes and other toxins, but also of particular consequence, to lower-quality environments on a daily basis at home, in school, on the job and in the neighborhood. The poor, especially the non-white poor, bear a disproportionate burden of exposure to lower-quality, unhealthy environmental conditions in this country.

We know that lifetime exposure to estrogen is a risk factor, so it is logical that if we have chemicals that are creating more estrogen, the risk goes up.

MEN CAN SUPPORT A WOMAN WITH BREAST CANCER

As we all know by now, October is Breast Cancer Awareness Month. What many of don't realize is that men get breast cancer too. But, most importantly, men have an important role when breast cancer strikes a woman in their life. Unfortunately, many men are clueless on how to be supportive during this critical period in a woman's life.

Every three minutes somewhere in the United States, a woman is told she has breast cancer.

That translates into one in every eight American women—or over 184,000 women in 2008. Breast cancer is one of those diseases where there isn't a simple formula for treatment.

Simply put, breast cancer is cancer that's found in breast tissue. If it spreads, those same breast cancer cells can establish themselves in lung, liver, bone, or brain tissue. Treatment is very individualized based on the woman's age, the size of the tumor, whether it's in the lymph nodes, and whether it's estrogen-receptor positive.

Cancer often forms in tissues of the breast, usually the ducts (tubes that carry milk to the nipple) and lobules (glands that make milk). It occurs in both men and women, although male breast cancer is rare.

Breast cancer begins in a cell, which divides and multiplies at an uncontrolled rate. A small clump of cancer cells are too tiny to be felt, so the earliest stages of breast cancer usually have no symptoms. A mammogram can detect cancer before a lump can be felt, which is why your annual screening mammogram is so important.

Unfortunately, for many men, the chances are high that at some point in the future, someone you know will develop the disease.

Most often men are left to figure out how to help their wife, mother, sister, daughter, aunt, cousin, colleague, or friend—not to mention how to deal with their own fears and frustrations—alone.

For many men, the biggest challenge is dealing with the fact that they can't "fix" this. The most important thing that a man must accept in his breast cancer journey with the woman he loves is that he cannot fix everything, but he must be there to listen, help, encourage and just be there for her-in other words love her even more.

Often, guys don't listen. They play the denial game. They don't want to admit how serious it is. They deal with their fears by working harder, staying at work, holing up in the den at home. They don't want to deal with their wife. They want her to work as much as she used to. But you can't pretend nothing has happened. You're not going to have the life you wanted to have. You're facing her surgery, chemotherapy, and/or radiation.

Men Can Support a Woman with Breast Cancer

One of the most helpful things you can do is gather information for her. She may well be feeling too confused and shocked to do it herself. But don't make that an excuse to give advice–just be a conduit of facts and let her think about those facts for herself.

When it comes to treatment, she may not necessarily make the same decision you would choose. She may opt for surgery when you would go the other way. Remember that it is her life, not yours, so support her decisions.

She will not be the only one who needs support.

Don't overstretch yourself, and be realistic about what you can do. Make sure that you yourself have help to get through your fear about her illness. Maintaining a proper diet makes a difference in helping you to have the energy, both physically and emotionally, to be an effective caregiver. Additionally, of course, stay off the alcohol and any other artificial means that you think will help you "escape" for a little while. Chemical-induced respites will not help in the long or short run.

As you have no doubt heard countless times: "Exercise! Make it part of your day like brushing your teeth. Even if it is for 15 minutes a day, do it. You and your family will reap the benefits that exercise and a proper diet will provide."

This doesn't mean that you have to turn into Jack Lelane, but you do need to pay special attention to your well being as well as your loved one. After all, if you are not there for yourself, how can you be there for her?

You really can't prevent breast cancer. A woman can live a healthy lifestyle: exercise; keep your weight in check, only a small amount of drinking, if any. That will help lower the risk. But the greatest risk factor for breast cancer is sex and age, neither of which is controllable.

And, though breast cancer can't be prevented, detecting it earlier can certainly lessen its seriousness. This means women being diligent about noticing any breast changes, and regular mammograms, once past the age of 40.

In recent years, there's been an explosion of life-saving treatment advances against breast cancer, bringing new hope and excitement. Instead of only one or two options, today there's an overwhelming menu of treatment choices that fight the complex mix of cells in each individual cancer.

Breast cancer, even when it's successfully treated, lingers in a woman's life for a long time.

Addressing a woman's cancer is a sensitive issue, but all men want to help. However, men often worry about not doing it "right". As a result, time passes, and to avoid doing it "wrong," we often don't do anything at all.

Keep these tips in mind:

- Listen without judging.
- Be as open as possible. If you're afraid, say so. If you want to cry, cry.
- Go to medical appointments with her whenever you can. If you can't go, make sure someone else does so she's not alone.
- Make her hospital stays more comfortable–get her the books or videos she likes and put personal touches in the room.
- Take care of yourself so you can be there for your family.

UNDERSTANDING CHEMOTHERAPY

Chemotherapy is the use of anti-cancer (cytotoxic) drugs to destroy cancer cells (including leukemia and lymphomas). There are over 50 different chemotherapy drugs and some are given on their own, but often several drugs may be combined (this is known as combination chemotherapy).

The type of treatment you are given for your cancer depends on many things, particularly the type of disease you have, where in the body it started, what the cancer cells look like under the microscope and how far they have spread, if at all.

Chemotherapy may be used alone to treat some types of cancer. Sometimes it can be used together with other types of treatment such as surgery, radiotherapy, immunotherapy, or a combination of these.

Chemotherapy drugs interfere with the ability of a cancer cell to divide and reproduce. As the drugs are carried in the blood, they can reach cancer cells all over the body. Healthy cells can repair the damage caused by chemotherapy but cancer cells cannot, and so they eventually die.

Chemotherapy has to be carefully planned so that it destroys more and more of the cancer cells during the course of treatment, but does not destroy the normal cells and tissues.

There are several reasons why a doctor may decide to have a person consider chemotherapy treatment:

- **To cure cancer**— with some types of cancer chemotherapy is likely to destroy all the cancer cells and cure the disease.
- **To reduce the chance of a cancer coming back** — chemotherapy may be given after surgery or radiotherapy so that if any cancer cells remain but are too small to see they can be destroyed by the chemotherapy.
- **To shrink a cancer and prolong life** — if a cure is not possible, chemotherapy may be given to shrink and control a cancer, or reduce the number of cancer cells, and try to prolong a good quality of life.
- Now, here is the part that causes most people to view chemotherapy as an undesirable option.

Yes, there are potential side effects, and before you or someone you love decides against it, make sure you fully understand the side effects. Then, and only then, can you weigh the pros and cons as they relate to a specific case.

Chemotherapy can reduce the number of blood cells produced by the bone marrow. Bone marrow is a spongy material that fills the bones and contains stem cells, which normally develop into the three different types of blood cell.

Understanding Chemotherapy

The cells produced by bone marrow:

1. White blood cells are essential for fighting infections.
2. Red blood cells contain hemoglobin to carry oxygen round the body.
3. Platelets help to clot the blood and prevent bleeding.

If the number of white cells in your blood is low you will be more likely to get an infection as there are fewer white cells to fight off bacteria.

Some chemotherapy drugs can cause feelings of sickness (nausea), or actually being sick (vomiting). Many people do not have any sickness with their chemotherapy. There are now very effective treatments to prevent and control sickness and this is much less of a problem than it was in the past. If you do feel sick, it will usually start from a few minutes to several hours after the chemotherapy, depending on the drugs given. The sickness may last for a few hours or, rarely, for several days.

Some chemotherapy drugs can reduce your appetite for a while. Some chemotherapy drugs can affect the lining of the digestive system and this may cause diarrhea for a few days. More rarely, some chemotherapy drugs can cause constipation.

If you have any diarrhea or constipation, or are worried about the effects of chemotherapy on your digestive system, see your doctor to discuss any problems you may have.

Chemotherapy can cause your taste to change; food may taste more salty, bitter or metallic. Normal taste will come back after the chemotherapy treatment finishes.

Hair loss is one of the most well-known side effects of chemotherapy.

Some drugs cause no hair loss or the amount of hair lost is so slight it is hardly noticeable. If hair loss happens it usually starts within a few weeks of beginning treatment, although very occasionally it can start within a few days. Underarm, body and pubic hair may be lost as well. Some drugs also cause loss of the eyelashes and eyebrows. If you do lose your hair as a result of chemotherapy, it will grow back once you have finished your treatment.

Some drugs can affect your skin. These may cause your skin to become dry or slightly discolored and may be made worse by swimming, especially if there is chlorine in the water. Any rashes should be reported to your doctor. The drugs may also make your skin more sensitive to sunlight, during and after the treatment. Protect your skin from the sun by wearing a hat, covering skin with loose clothing and using sunscreen cream on any exposed areas.

Your nails may grow more slowly and you may notice white lines appearing across them. False nails or nail varnish can disguise white lines. Your nails may also become more brittle and flaky.

Some chemotherapy drugs can affect the nerves in the hands and feet. This can cause tingling or numbness, or a sensation of pins and needles. This is known as peripheral neuropathy. Some drugs can cause feelings of anxiety and restlessness, dizziness, sleeplessness or headaches. Some people also find it hard to concentrate on anything.

Some of our chemotherapy medications are derived from herbs. For example, the Vinca family–Vincristine, Vinblastine — are derived from the herb periwinkle. Taxol is also from a plant/tree in the northern rain forest. For those on chemotherapy, medication, herbs are not without some side effects. It is therefore always very important to keep your medical team informed of what supplements you are taking.

THE DANGERS OF HIGH BLOOD PRESSURE

Untreated high blood pressure increases the risk of heart disease, stroke, problems with blood vessels and blood flow, kidney and eye problems, and early death. It is estimated that 1 of 3 American adults has high blood pressure or hypertension.

High blood pressure is often called the 'silent killer' because it usually has no noticeable warning signs or symptoms until other serious problems arise. Therefore, many people with high blood pressure do not know that they have it. High blood pressure is a major risk factor for heart disease, the leading cause of death in the United States. It can lead to hardened or stiffened arteries, which causes a decrease of blood flow to the heart muscle and other parts of the body. Reduced blood to the heart muscle can lead to angina or to a heart attack.

Blood pressure is the force of blood against the artery walls. It is often written or stated as two numbers. The first or top number represents the pressure when the heart contracts. This is called systolic pressure. The second or bottom number represents the pressure when the heart rests between beats. This is called diastolic pressure.

High blood pressure is a major risk factor for heart failure, a serious condition where the heart cannot pump enough blood for the body's needs. It is also the major risk factor for stroke, which is the third leading cause of death in the United States. A stroke may be caused by a rupture or blockage of an artery that supplies blood and oxygen to the brain.

In addition, high blood pressure can result in damage to the eyes, including blindness. The blood vessels in the eyes can rupture or burst from high blood pressure leading to impairment of sight.

High blood pressure can also result in kidney disease and kidney failure. The kidneys filter wastes from fluids in the body. High blood pressure can thicken and narrow the blood vessels of the kidneys, resulting in less fluid being filtered and wastes building up in the body. Also, diseases of the kidney can be a cause of high blood pressure.

If you have diabetes, you are at least twice as likely as someone who does not have diabetes to have heart disease or a stroke. People with diabetes also tend to develop heart disease or have strokes at an earlier age than other people. If you are middle-aged and have type 2 diabetes, some studies suggest that your chance of having a heart attack is as high as someone without diabetes who has already had one heart attack.

People with diabetes who have already had one heart attack run an even greater risk of having a second one. In addition, heart attacks in people with diabetes are more serious and more likely to result in death. High blood glucose levels over time can lead to increased deposits of fatty materials on the insides of the blood vessel walls. These deposits may affect blood flow, increasing the chance of clogging and hardening of blood vessels (atherosclerosis).

A stroke results when the blood supply to the brain is suddenly cut off, which can occur when a blood vessel in the brain or neck is blocked or bursts. Brain cells are then deprived of oxygen and die. Fatty deposits or blood clots—jelly-like clumps of blood cells—that narrow or block one of the blood vessels in the brain or neck cause most strokes. A blood clot may stay where it formed or can travel within the body. People with diabetes are at increased risk for strokes caused by blood clots. A stroke may also be caused by a bleeding blood vessel in the brain., called an aneurysm, which is a break in a blood vessel can occur as a result of high blood pressure or a weak spot in a blood vessel wall.

There are several types of medications that are used to treat high blood pressure. Frequently, more than one type will be used. It is important to take these as prescribed. High blood pressure medicines fall into one of these types:

- **Diuretics** work in the kidney and flush excess water and sodium from the body. They are sometimes called "water pills."
- **Beta–blockers** reduce nerve impulses to the heart and blood vessels that make the heart beat slower and with less force.
- **Angiotensin–converting enzyme (ACE) inhibitors** cause the blood vessels to relax. ACE inhibitors prevent the formation of a hormone called angiotensin II, which normally causes the blood vessels to narrow.
- **Angiotensin antagonists** shield the blood vessels from angiotensin II. As a result, the vessels become wider.

- **Calcium channel blockers** prevent calcium from entering the muscle cells of the heart and blood vessels. This causes the blood vessels to relax.
- **Alpha–blockers** reduce nerve impulses to the blood vessels, which allows the blood to pass more easily.
- **Alpha–beta–blockers** work the same way as alpha-blockers but also slow the heartbeat, as beta–blockers do. As a result, less blood is pumped through the vessels.
- **Nervous system inhibitors** relax blood vessels by controlling nerve impulses. This causes the blood vessels to become wider.
- **Vasodilators** directly open the blood vessels by relaxing the muscle in the vessel walls.

It is important to keep in mind that high blood pressure can be prevented or controlled through lifestyle changes and with medications when needed.

KIDNEY DISEASE
LEADS TO DIALYSIS

Even though there is no single cause of chronic kidney disease, any condition or disease that damages blood vessels or other structures in the kidneys can lead to kidney disease. The most common causes of chronic kidney disease are:

- Diabetes. Diabetes causes about 35% of all chronic kidney disease. High blood sugar levels caused by diabetes damage blood vessels in the kidneys. If the blood sugar level remains high, this damage gradually reduces the function of the kidneys.

- High blood pressure (hypertension). High blood pressure causes another 30% of all kidney disease. Because blood pressure often rises with chronic kidney disease, high blood pressure may further damage kidney function even when another medical condition initially caused the disease.

Other conditions that can damage the kidneys and cause chronic kidney disease include:

- Kidney diseases and infections, or a kidney problem you were born with.
- Having a narrowed or blocked renal artery. The renal artery carries blood to the kidneys.
- Having an enlarged prostate gland, kidney stones, or a tumor that keeps urine from flowing out of the kidneys.
- Lead poisoning.
- Long-term use of medicines that can damage the kidneys. Examples include pain medicines, like acetaminophen (such as Tylenol) and ibuprofen (such as Advil), and certain antibiotics

Your kidneys play a key role in keeping your blood pressure in a healthy range, and blood pressure, in turn, can affect the health of your kidneys.

High blood pressure makes your heart work harder and, over time, can damage blood vessels throughout your body. If the blood vessels in your kidneys are damaged, they may stop removing wastes and extra fluid from your body. The extra fluid in your blood vessels may then raise blood pressure even more. It's a dangerous cycle.

About 30 percent of people with diabetes will go on to develop kidney failure, while even more may be at risk of premature death from cardiovascular disease. Eighty to ninety percent of patients with type 2 diabetes also have hypertension, a major risk factor for diabetic kidney disease.

Kidney Disease leads to Dialysis

The kidneys are responsible for filtering waste products from the blood. Dialysis is a procedure that is a substitute for many of the normal duties of the kidneys. Another major duty of the kidney is to remove the waste products that the body produces throughout the day. As the body functions, the cells use energy. The operation of the cells produces waste products that must be removed from the body. When these waste products are not removed adequately, they build up in the body. An elevation of waste products, as measured in the blood, is called "azotemia." When waste products accumulate they can cause a sick feeling throughout the body called "uremia."

Dialysis is a method of removing toxic substances (impurities or wastes) from the blood when the kidneys are unable to do so. Once the kidney function drops to a certain level, dialysis becomes necessary. In the United States, there are over 200,000 people who use dialysis techniques on an ongoing basis. Dialysis helps the body by performing the functions of failed kidneys. The kidney has many roles. An essential job of the kidney is to regulate the body's fluid balance. It does this by adjusting the amount of urine that is excreted on a daily basis. On hot days, the body sweats more. Thus, less water needs to be excreted through the kidneys. On cold days, the body sweats less. Thus, urine output needs to be greater in order to maintain the proper balance within the body. It is the kidney's job to regulate fluid balance by adjusting urine output.

Diseases that increase your chance of developing kidney failure are diabetes, high blood pressure, heart failure, obesity, and long-term kidney disease (chronic renal insufficiency). If you have any of these conditions, take extra precautions when starting new medicines. Commonly used medicines, such as aspirin and ibuprofen (nonsteroidal anti-inflammatory drugs), can make kidney function worse in people who already have impaired kidney function, diabetes, high blood pressure, or heart failure.

Do what you can to reduce the chances of kidney failure. Some basic tips are:

- **Maintain your weight** at a level close to normal. Choose fruits, vegetables, grains, and low-fat dairy foods.
- **Limit your daily sodium (salt) intake** to 2,000 milligrams or lower if you already have high blood pressure. Read <u>nutrition</u> labels on packaged foods to learn how much sodium is in one serving. Keep a sodium diary.
- **Get plenty of exercise,** which means at least 30 minutes of moderate activity, such as walking, most days of the week.
- **Avoid consuming too much alcohol.** Men should limit consumption to two drinks (two 12-ounce servings of beer or two 5-ounce servings of wine or two 1.5-ounce servings of "hard" liquor) a day. Women should have no more than a single serving on a given day because <u>metabolic</u> differences make women more susceptible to the effects of alcohol.
- **Limit your caffeine intake.** This includes sodas, chocolate, as well as coffees and teas.

If you have kidney damage, you should keep your blood pressure below 130/80.

Remember, I'm not a doctor. I just sound like one.

Take good care of yourself and live the best life possible.

CHOLESTEROL IS IMPORTANT

A membrane made largely of cholesterol, fat and protein covers every cell in your body. Without adequate cholesterol, cell membranes become too fluid, and not rigid enough. If your cell membranes suddenly became totally devoid of cholesterol, your cells would explode from their internal water pressure like over-filled water balloons. Brain cells are particularly rich in cholesterol, the brain being about 7% cholesterol.

One of cholesterol's most important functions is to serve as the basic raw material from which your body makes many major hormones, including testosterone, estrogen, progesterone, cortisone and aldosterone. Without these first three hormones you would have no sex life; without cortisone your body could not cope with stress; and without aldosterone your body could not properly balance your sodium and water levels.

Large amounts of cholesterol are found in the skin, where it makes the skin highly resistant to the absorption of water-soluble toxins. The skin's cholesterol also helps hold water in the body, so that loss of water through skin evaporation is only about half to one pint daily, instead of the four to ten quarts of water which would be lost if not for skin cholesterol. Even your solid bones would be hollow and brittle, if not for cholesterol.

As much as 70% of the body's cholesterol is used by the liver to produce bile salts, used during food digestion to emulsify fats.

Your liver makes not only cholesterol, but also two main carrier molecules, LDL and HDL, which bind with cholesterol. Without help them, cholesterol could not travel through the blood stream. LDL (Low Density Lipoprotein) carries cholesterol out to all the tissues in the body, where it may be used for various functions, including production and repair of cell membranes, as well as hormone production. Unfortunately LDL-bound cholesterol also tends to stick to damaged artery linings, where it may accumulate, eventually plugging up the arteries and blocking blood flow. This is why LDL cholesterol often is referred to as the "bad" cholesterol.

About one-fourth to one-third of blood cholesterol is carried by high-density lipoprotein (HDL). HDL cholesterol is known as "good" cholesterol, because high levels of HDL seem to protect against heart attack. Triglyceride is a form of fat made in the body. Elevated triglycerides can be due to overweight/obesity, physical inactivity, cigarette smoking, excess alcohol consumption and a diet very high in carbohydrates.

Blood cholesterol levels should ideally be under 200. However, it is also important to remember that the connection between blood cholesterol levels and heart disease is a statistical phenomenon, only truly accurate when applied to estimating heart health risks of large groups of suffer a heart attack, while 15% of all fatal heart attacks will occur in people whose cholesterol were under the current "magic" number of 200.

The following lifestyle measures can be helpful in lowering total and LDL cholesterol, while raising HDL cholesterol.

- Regular aerobic exercise: jogging, brisk walking, bicycling, etc.
- Reducing dietary saturated fats and simple sugars, the two foodstuffs your liver is an expert at turning into blood cholesterol.
- No smoking and minimal alcohol intake.
- A high fiber diet: whole grains, beans, peas, lentils and fresh vegetables.
- Using olive oil as the primary salad and cooking oil, or flaxseed oil. These oils are high in monosaturated fats, which contribute to the elevation of HDL and the apparent reduction of LDL cholesterol.
- Maintaining proper weight. This is best done by exercise and low-fat foods.
- Frequent consumption of fish that are rich in the fatty acids EPA and DHA, such as sardines, salmon or cod, or of EPA/DHA rich fish oil capsules.
- Avoid animal foods fried in oil.

SUGGESTED NUTRIENTS FOR HEALTHY HEARTS:

Coenzyme Q 10 (CoQ10)- an essential nutrient needed for production of energy in every cell. It normally diminishes as we age which makes supplementation wise, even in healthy people. CoQ10 provides many benefits; a few of those being immune system enhancement, antiaging, circulatory support, tissue oxygenation, antihistamine properties, tumor reduction in cancer, strengthens the heart muscle, and improves blood pressure, treats gum disease, and more.

Vitamin C- Vitamin C helps rebuild collagen for arterial wall integrity and prevention of plaque build-up. It helps reduce inflammation in the body which lowers CRP levels. CRP levels are an indicator of inflammation in the body.

Grape Seed Extract- It promotes healthy circulation and protects cells from free radical damage.. It has anti-inflammatory, anti-viral, and anti-bacterial properties. Grape seed extract is one of only a few that can penetrate the blood brain barrier to protect the brain and nerve tissue.

Omega-3/6 Fatty Acids. They help reduce heart beat irregularities and blood clots, and help to normalize blood pressure.

B Vitamins- a combo of B_6, B_{12}, and Folic Acid, which help reduce homocysteine- a known risk factor for heart disease.

Vitamin E- It's been said that "E" is for Everything. It not only protects LDL cholesterol from oxidation, but protects ALL organ tissues from oxidation.

Magnesium- Helps control heart rhythm and blood pressure, and protects the lining of arteries.

Alpha-lipoic Acid (ALA)- Has powerful antioxidant properties. It is a valuable free radical scavenger since it is both water AND fat soluble. It, inhibits inflammation and plaque build-up, and works with magnesium to control blood pressure and reduce insulin sensitivity in diabetics.

Green Tea Extract- has antioxidant, antibacterial, and antiviral activity. It lowers LDL cholesterol, prevents clotting, and also plays a role in Cancer prevention.

HEART FAILURE

=====

Heart failure does not mean the heart has stopped working. Rather, it means that the heart's pumping power is weaker than normal. With heart failure, blood moves through the heart and body at a slower rate, and pressure in the heart increases. As a result, the heart cannot pump enough oxygen and nutrients to meet the body's needs. The chambers of the heart respond by stretching to hold more blood to pump through the body. This helps to keep the blood moving, but in time, the heart muscle walls weaken and are unable to pump as strongly. As a result, the kidneys often respond by causing the body to retain fluid (water) and sodium. If fluid builds up in the arms, legs, ankles, feet, lungs or other organs, the body becomes congested, and congestive heart failure is the term used to describe the condition.

Heart failure is caused by many conditions that damage the heart muscle, including:

- **Coronary artery disease:** CAD, a disease of the arteries that supply blood and oxygen to the heart, causes decreased blood flow to the heart muscle. If the arteries become blocked, the heart becomes starved for oxygen and nutrients.

- **Heart Attack:** A heart attack may occur when a coronary artery becomes suddenly blocked, stopping the flow of blood to the heart muscle and damaging it. All or part of the heart muscle becomes cut off from its supply of oxygen. A heart attack can damage the heart muscle, resulting in a scarred area that does not function properly.

- **Cardiomyopathy:** Damage to the heart muscle from causes other than artery or blood flow problems, such as from infections or alcohol or drug abuse.

- **Conditions that overwork the heart:** High blood pressure (hypertension), valve disease, thyroid disease, kidney disease, diabetes or heart defects present at birth can all cause heart failure. In addition, heart failure can occur when several diseases or conditions are present at once.

The symptoms of Heart Failure can include:

- **Congested lungs:** Fluid back up in the lungs can cause shortness of breath with exercise or difficulty breathing at rest or when lying flat in bed. Lung congestion also causes a dry, hacking cough or wheezing.

- **Fluid and water retention:** Less blood to your kidneys causes fluid and water retention, resulting in swollen ankles, legs and abdomen (called edema) and weight gain. Symptoms may cause an increased need to urinate during the night. Bloating in your stomach may cause a loss of appetite or nausea.

- **Dizziness, fatigue and weakness:** Less blood to your major organs and muscles makes you feel tired and weak. Less blood to the brain can cause dizziness or confusion.
- **Rapid or irregular heartbeats:** The heart beats faster to pump enough blood to the body. This causes a fast or irregular heartbeat.

If you have heart failure, you may have one or all of these symptoms or you may have none of them. There are some things you can do yourself to make things better:

- Stop smoking or chewing tobacco.
- Reach and maintain your healthy weight.
- Control high blood pressure, cholesterol levels and diabetes.
- Exercise regularly.
- Do not drink alcohol.

There are also some specific things to do that can lesson the symptoms:

- **Maintain fluid balance.** Remember, the more fluid you carry in your blood vessels, the harder your heart must work to pump excess fluid through your body. Limiting your fluid intake to less than a half-gallon per day will help decrease the workload of your heart and prevent symptoms from recurring.
- **Limit how much salt (sodium) you eat.** Sodium is found naturally in many foods we eat. It is also added for flavoring or to make food last longer. If you follow a low-sodium diet, you

should have less fluid retention, less swelling and breathe easier.

- **Monitor your weight and lose weight if needed.** Learn what your "dry" or "ideal" weight is. This is your weight without extra water (fluid). Your goal is to keep your weight within four pounds of your dry weight. Weigh yourself at the same time each day, preferably in the morning, in similar clothing, after urinating but before eating, and on the same scale. Record your weight in a diary or calendar. If you gain two pounds in one day or five pounds in one week, call your doctor.

- **Take your medications as prescribed.** Medications are used to improve your heart's ability to pump blood, decrease stress on your heart, decrease the progression of heart failure and prevent fluid retention. Many heart failure medications are used to decrease the release of harmful hormones. These drugs will cause your blood vessels to dilate or relax (thereby lowering your blood pressure).

By the way, there are some definite medications you should avoid:

- Non-steroidal anti-inflammatory drugs such as Tylenol or Motrin
- Most antiarrhythmic agents
- Most calcium channel blockers
- Some nutritional supplements and growth hormone therapies
- Antacids that contain sodium (salt)
- Decongestants such as Sudafed (they make your heart work harder)

If you are taking any of these medications, discuss them with your doctor.

It is important to know the names of your medications, what they are used for and how often and at what times you take them. Keep a list of your medications and bring them with you to each of your doctor visits. **Never stop taking your medications without discussing it with your doctor.** Even if you have no symptoms, your medications decrease the work of your heart so that it can pump more effectively.

STRESS, HEART ATTACKS, AND STROKES

=====

It's important to learn how to recognize when your stress levels are out of control. The most dangerous thing about stress is how easily it can creep up on you. You get used to it. It starts to feels familiar – even normal. You don't notice how much it's affecting you, even as it takes a heavy toll.

The signs and symptoms of stress overload can be almost anything. Stress affects the mind, body, and behavior in many ways, and everyone experiences stress differently.

A driving analogy best describes the three most common ways people respond when they're overwhelmed by stress:

- **Foot on the gas** – An angry or agitated stress response. You're heated, keyed up, and overly emotional.
- **Foot on the brake** – A withdrawn or depressed stress response. You shut down, space out, and show very little energy or emotion.

Stress, Heart Attacks, and Strokes

- **Foot on both** – A tense and frozen stress response. You "freeze" under pressure and can't do anything. You look paralyzed, but under the surface you're extremely agitated.

The rise in heart rate and blood pressure during stress may increase your heart's need for oxygen while simultaneously reducing its supply. The heart's arteries (coronary arteries) usually dilate during stress in order to deliver blood to needed body parts as quickly as possible. If you suffer from atherosclerosis ("hardening of the arteries"), your coronary arteries may be unable to dilate sufficiently under stress.

Stress may promote several of the factors that lead to blood clots (thrombosis) of the arteries leading to the heart (coronary arteries), or even a massive stroke!

Although men and women have strokes at about the same rate, women more often die of strokes than do men. Blacks are more likely to have strokes than are people of other races.

The stress that you feel all the time is working against your body and causing you to have many physical and emotional problems at the same time.

Another problem with stress is it will cause high blood pressure. When you get worked up and upset over things you will start to feel your blood start to rise and your heart will pound. This feeling is making your bodywork harder than it has to. This is something that may cause you to feel bad inside and out, and give you more stress than what you already had.

Many of us out there feel the pressures of daily life. This can be work related or family related. There are so many things in life that cause us a great deal of stress and worry.

The key is to not let these things bother us too much. When we get worked up and upset over everything in life, we are only adding to the problems that we have and this is certainly not good for the heart.

Many times a person with too much stress in their life will have a stroke and then it is too late to do anything about it.

When you or someone you know is so stressed out with their life, they need to find a release so the stress won't take over and cause a stroke. Men with greater work-related stress were found to have an increased risk of accelerated development of carotid artery (a main supply route to the brain) atherosclerosis, which can lead to strokes. People who feel stressed out week-in-week-out had a significant increased risk of fatal stroke.

Certain chronic responses to stress have been associated with heart disease. Two of these responses are hostility and cynicism. If you are chronically hostile and/or cynical, you are more likely to manifest larger increases in heart rate, blood pressure, and stress hormones in response to non-social stressors than are individuals with low hostility.

Numerous surveys confirm that occupational pressures are far and away the leading source of stress for American adults and that job stress has escalated progressively over the past four decades. This is becoming even more relevant in the times we are living.

Two specific areas that are impacting many of my friends are:

- Management Style—Lack of participation by workers in decision-making; poor communication in the organization; lack of company policies that take employees' family and personal obligations into consideration.

Stress, Heart Attacks, and Strokes

- Concerns About Employment Or Career–Job insecurity and lack of opportunity for advancement, or promotion; rapid changes for which workers are unprepared due to unanticipated downsizing, mergers and hostile acquisitions.

In many instances, we create our own stress that contributes to coronary disease by smoking and other faulty lifestyles or because of dangerous traits like excess anger, hostility, aggressiveness, time urgency, inappropriate competitiveness and preoccupation with work. These are characteristic of Type A coronary prone behavior, now recognized to be as significant a risk factor for heart attacks and coronary events as cigarette consumption, elevated cholesterol and blood pressure.

Stress is an unavoidable consequence of life but there are some stresses you can do something about and others that you can't hope to avoid or control. The trick is in learning to distinguish between the two. The best way to accomplish this is in learning how to correct faulty perceptions and develop a better sense of control over your activities at work as well as at home. This will not only improve your quality of life but also help protect you from heart attacks and strokes. You will start to feel better knowing that you are doing everything you need to do so that you are not faces with the high blood pressure and stress and stroke.

SUDDEN
CARDIAC ARREST

The most common underlying reason for patients to die suddenly from cardiac arrest is coronary heart disease. Most cardiac arrests that lead to sudden death occur when the electrical impulses in the diseased heart become rapid (ventricular tachycardia) or chaotic (ventricular fibrillation) or both. This irregular heart rhythm (arrhythmia) causes the heart to suddenly stop beating.

The heart has an internal electrical system that controls the rhythm of the heartbeat. Problems can cause abnormal heart rhythms, called arrhythmias. There are many types of arrhythmia. During an arrhythmia, the heart can beat too fast, too slow, or it can stop beating. Sudden cardiac arrest occurs when the heart develops an arrhythmia that causes it to stop beating. This is different than a heart attack, where the heart usually continues to beat but blood flow to the heart is blocked.

There are many possible causes of cardiac arrest. They include coronary heart disease, heart attack, electrocution, drowning, or choking.

There may not be a known cause to the cardiac arrest.

What is clear is that there are ways to lower one's risk of sudden cardiac death, these include healthy diet, exercising regularly, not smoking and taking aspirins. The trouble, though, is that patients often don't think they're at serious risk until they are actually experiencing an attack. In about a third of all sudden deaths due to coronary disease, the first sign that anything was wrong was death itself.

A sudden cardiac arrest is, of course, unexpected, but the process that causes it may begin many years before. In middle-aged men, it's virtually always caused by degeneration in the wall of a coronary artery.

The sad fact is that the majority of acute heart attacks are associated with "non-significant" plaques. These plaques may suddenly rupture, which quickly leads to the formation of a blood clot. The blood clot acutely occludes the coronary artery, causing a heart attack.

Brain death and permanent death start to occur in just 4 to 6 minutes after someone experiences cardiac arrest. Cardiac arrest can be reversed if it's treated within a few minutes with an electric shock to the heart to restore a normal heartbeat. This process is called defibrillation. A victim's chances of survival are reduced by 7 to 10 percent with every minute that passes without CPR and defibrillation. Few attempts at resuscitation succeed after 10 minutes.

According to NCHS Data Warehouse, 325,000 coronary heart disease deaths occur out-of-hospital or in hospital emergency departments annually.

The term "massive heart attack" is often wrongly used in the media to describe sudden death. The term "heart attack" refers to death of heart muscle tissue due to the loss of blood supply, not necessarily resulting in a cardiac arrest or the death of the heart attack victim. A heart attack may cause cardiac arrest and sudden cardiac death, but the terms aren't the same.

Sudden death in people under age 35, often due to hidden heart defects or overlooked heart abnormalities, is rare. These sudden deaths often occur during physical activity, such as a sporting event.

Millions of elementary, high school and college athletes compete every year without incident. Still, when sudden cardiac arrest or sudden cardiac death in a young person is due to a heart abnormality, it's often triggered by physical activity. Fortunately, if you're at risk of sudden death, there are screening tests to see if you have a heart defect and precautions you can take to protect your heart.

Cardiac arrest is obviously a serious medical emergency. The mortality (death rate) from cardiac arrest can be decreased by providing immediate CPR and prompt defibrillation. Many public places are now equipped with automated external defibrillators (AEDs) that allow laypersons to provide emergency defibrillation in case of cardiac arrest.

DIABETIC
NEUROPATHY

Today, I ran into a good friend I've known since college. In addition to being happy to see him, he stunned me with two shocking facts.

The first was that this year marks the 40th anniversary of us entering college. The second was that he was diabetic, and experiencing the symptoms of diabetic neuropathy.

Not only was he in almost constant pain, he had even resorted to sleeping with his sneakers on, in order to have enough pressure on his feet to quiet down the nerves.

We all know that diabetes can be a devastating condition, but what many don't realize is that over time diabetes can lead to blindness, kidney failure, and nerve damage.

DPN (diabetic peripheral neuropathy) is a serious condition that results from damage to nerves due to prolonged exposure to high amounts of glucose in the bloodstream as a result of diabetes. It often results in pain or numbness in the feet, but also manifests itself in intense pain often described as aching, tingling, burning and numbness, but because DPN damages nerve fibers, virtually any nerve in the body can be affected. The feet and toes are commonly affected early in the course of a generalized neuropathy.

The term "peripheral" means that the disease is occurring to nerve tissue outside the brain and spinal cord. This includes injury of nerves to muscles (motor nerves), nerves from the skin (sensory nerves), and/or nerves to the gut and other internal organs (autonomic nerves).

More than half of all diabetics suffer from DPN. In the U.S., African Americans are 1.6 times more likely to have diabetes than non-Hispanic whites, and Hispanic/Latino Americans are 1.8 times more likely to have diabetes than non-Hispanic whites.

The leading cause of amputations in the U.S., DPN causes as much as 40 to 60 percent of lower extremity amputations, with the African American, Latino and Native American diabetic populations at twice the rate of the diabetic white population.

In the United States, more than 50,000 diabetes-related amputations are performed each year, but comprehensive foot care programs can reduce amputation rates by 45 to 85 percent.

It is helpful to understand the different types of nerves that can be involved. The sensory nerves send messages back to the brain about various sensations, such as temperature, pain, and movement. Motor nerves send signals from the brain to the muscles to tell them to move. Autonomic nerves are involuntary, and control such things as heart rate, smooth muscles, and the function of glands. Diabetic neuropathy can cause pain in the nerves of both legs or partial or complete loss of feeling, particularly in lower limbs. The pain is often worse in bed at night.

Diabetic Neuropathy

Diabetic peripheral neuropathy is the most common neuropathy in the United States and the world. It is estimated that there are 15-20 million cases of diabetic neuropathy in the United States. Given the size of this problem, isn't it strange that more people do not know about it? Diabetic neuropathy contributes to the incidence of lower limb amputations in diabetic patients because diabetics are less likely to perceive a wound in their feet or legs.

Since diabetic neuropathies are a family of nerve disorders caused by diabetes, some people with diabetes can, over time, develop nerve damage throughout the body. Some people with nerve damage have no symptoms. Neuropathic pain can feel like burning, prickling, tingling, aching, stabbing, pins and needles, shooting, and even like an electrical current "buzz." The most common type of neuropathic pain occurs on both sides of the body, as in both legs and feet, or both hands. Neuropathic pain can come and go or it can continue for a long time. Nerve problems can occur in every organ system, including the digestive tract, heart, and sex organs.

About 60 to 70 percent of people with diabetes have some form of neuropathy. People with diabetes can develop nerve problems at any time, but risk rises with age and longer duration of diabetes. The highest rates of neuropathy are among people who have had diabetes for at least 25 years. Diabetic neuropathies also appear to be more common in people who have problems controlling their blood glucose, also called blood sugar, as well as those with high levels of blood fat and blood pressure and those who are overweight.

As with any medical problem, the proper diagnosis of a peripheral neuropathy requires that a physician take a history and perform a physical examination. The history must include a review of any currently prescribed medications because some medications can cause a peripheral neuropathy.

In some cases, diabetic neuropathy can be prevented. Patients who follow their recommended self-care program are less likely to develop diabetic neuropathy. Here is what you can do to prevent nerve damage:

- Keep your blood glucose as close to normal as you can.
- Limit the amount of alcohol you drink.
- Don't smoke.
- Take care of your feet
- Tell your doctor about any problems you have with
  1. your hands, arms, feet, or legs
  2. your stomach, bowels, or bladder
- Also tell your doctor if you
  1. have problems when you have sex
  2. cannot always tell when your blood glucose is too low
  3. feel dizzy when you go from lying down to sitting or standing

No one knows exactly what causes diabetic neuropathy, but studies have shown that people whose blood sugar levels are not well controlled are more likely to develop it. Research also suggests that about half of persons who have had diabetes for a long time (more than 25 years) will develop some type of neuropathy. People with diabetes who smoke and drink alcohol are more likely to develop neuropathy.

Pain medications can help, especially if taken at regular times throughout the day. Waiting until the pain becomes severe before taking medication is not as effective as taking regularly scheduled doses. Your health care provider will prescribe pain medication after reviewing your medical condition. Depending on the type and level of pain, your health care provider might recommend an over-the-counter pain medication or a prescription drug.

Diabetic neuropathic pain can be prevented in some cases and improved in most cases.

OBESITY AS A GATEWAY DISEASE

Ever heard of the gateway drug theory? According to this theory, the habitual use of less dangerous drugs may lead to a future risk of using more dangerous hard drugs. Based on this theory then, people who frequently use marijuana are more likely to use harder drugs, such as cocaine or heroin, in the future. In this sense, it is believed that, marijuana serves as a gateway drug.

The theory suggests that, all other things being equal, an adolescent who uses any one drug is more likely to use another drug. In practice, early introduction to substance use for adolescents is often through tobacco and/or alcohol. These two drugs are considered the first "gate" for most adolescents. Under this hypothesis, tobacco, alcohol, and marijuana are all considered "gateway drugs," preceding the use of one another and of illicit drugs.

Obesity is not just being overweight but a disease in itself. Just as you need a treatment for any other disease and you need to consult a doctor for your sickness, similarly obesity also needs a proper medical attention.

Obesity is not only just about overeating and a flabby body. In fact Obesity is the gateway to a whole range of health problems. Actually obese people should not be an object of laughter but to be worried and cared for. We first have to understand that which kind of people fall into the category of obesity. Obesity is generally calculated according to the BMI index of a person's body. BMI stands for the body mass index of a person. BMI is calculated on the basis of the height of a person in pounds divided by the square of his height in meters. If a person's BMI is 30 or more than 30, then he can be called an obese person. Obese people are prone to developing several cardio-vascular diseases, including high cholesterol leading to cardiac arrest, hypertension or high blood pressure, diabetes, arthritis and pain in the various joints of the body, to name just a few.

Obesity seems to be the same as death. It has created a do or die kind of situation for the people suffering from it. If one does not take any measures to control the increasing body weight he or she is bound to fall prey to this dreadful disease.

Obesity in general terms means being highly overweight. Obesity, in the current scenario is not looked just as being overweight but as a serious disease that can cause fatal health conditions like heart attack or even cancer. Overweight or obesity is caused by accumulation of fats in the body over a period of time. This happens due to consumption of more and more calories on one hand, and burning less of it on the other hand.

Besides having these health problems, obese people find it difficult to adjust themselves in society. They develop stress and can even fall into depression. Hence, obesity is such an alarming condition that if ignored, it can lead to grave consequences.

Major causes of the obesity are:

- Overeating
- Poor eating lifestyle/Frequency of eating
- Lack of exercise
- Genetics (family history/background of obesity)
- Medical illnesses
- Medications
- Stressful life events or changes
- Low self-esteem
- Diseases (depression or other emotional problems)

Obese people have a 50 to 100% larger risk of death from all causes as compared to normal-weight people. Most people comprehend that glut fat is harmful, but the problem is where the fat is distributed. People with apple-shaped bodies (fattest in the belly) have a greater jeopardy of heart disease and diabetes than those with pear shapes (fattest in the hips, buttocks, and thighs).

Obesity in adults often has its roots in childhood. In the developed world, obesity in children is growing at a frighteningly fast rate. There are more obese children now than ever before. Many people believe that parents are letting their carelessness with their own diets spill over into their children's lives.

The primary treatment for obesity is dieting and physical exercise. A sedentary lifestyle plays a significant role in obesity. Worldwide there has been a large shift towards less physically demanding work, and currently at least 60% of the world's population gets insufficient exercise. This is primarily due to increasing use of mechanized transportation and a greater prevalence of labor-saving technology in the home.

In both children and adults, there is an association between television viewing time and the risk of obesity. A 2008 study found that 63 of 73 studies (86%) showed an increased rate of childhood obesity with increased media exposure; with rates increasing proportionally to time spent watching television.

Many people are concerned in our culture that far too many children are becoming overweight and in some cases obese. Obesity in children is a growing trend and this trend can have significant negative affects on a child's physical as well as mental health.

Many children are eating too much or eating the wrong kinds of food causing them to become obese. Part of the problem is processed food and fast food. Many times all a child needs is to have a balanced and healthy diet available for each meal. Unfortunately with our hectic lives it is far easier to get a meal at the local fast food restaurant then cook a healthy dinner or lunch at home. Many children are eating burgers and fries when they should be eating more fruits and vegetables. Another problem is processed foods. Many children have grown accustomed to chips, chocolate bars and junk food. Most of the times a child only wants to eat something that tastes good and they don't care if it is nutritious or not. This is a time that a parent must be strict with their child and explain to them that junk food on a regular basis is not healthy. Parents are sometimes enabling their child to eat unhealthy food, which can cause obesity.

Gateway drugs are by no means as immediately dangerous as the harder stuff, but they nevertheless cause problems in the long run. Obesity is just as much a contributor to deadly diseases. Save the children...

HEALTH RISKS
OF BELLY FAT

━━━━━━━━━━

Are you one of the many people who think you can get rid of that "belly" by strengthening your abdominal muscles? Think again. You can do sit-ups 'til the cows come home, but nothing short of actual weight loss will do the trick.

It would help if we had a better understanding of those bigger waistlines as we age.

Of course it is on a practical level the result of gaining weight. But ultimately the problem is body fat.

There are two types of fat that you have in your abdominal area. The first type that covers up your abdominal area is called subcutaneous fat and lies directly beneath the skin and on top of the abdominal muscles.

The second type of fat that you have in your abdominal area is called visceral fat, and that lies deeper in the abdomen beneath your muscle and surrounding your organs.

Visceral fat also plays a role in giving certain men that "beer belly" appearance where their abdomen protrudes excessively but at the same time, also feels sort of hard if you push on it. The average American has about 30 billion fat cells: each of them is filled with greasy substances called lipids. When you pump doughnuts, potato chips, and candy bars into your system, those fat cells can expand-up to 1,000 times their original size. But a fat cell can get only so big; once it reaches its physical limit, it starts to behave like a long-running sitcom. It creates spin-offs, leaving you with two or more fat cells for the price of one. Only problem: Fat cells have a no-return policy. Once you have a fat cell, you're stuck with it- they never go away. So as you grow fatter and double the number of fat cells in your body, you also double the difficulty you'll have losing the lipids inside them.

Many of us tend to store fat in our bellies, and that's where the health dangers of excess weight begin. Abdominal fat doesn't just sit there and do nothing; it's active. It functions like a separate organ, releasing substances that can be harmful to your body. For instance, it releases free fatty acids that impair your ability to break down the hormone insulin (too much insulin in your system can lead to diabetes). Fat also secretes substances that increase your risk of heart attacks and strokes, as well as the stress hormone cortisol (high levels of cortisol are also associated with diabetes and obesity as well as with high blood pressure). Abdominal fat bears the blame for many health problems because it resides within striking distance of your heart, liver, and other organs pressing on them, feeding them poisons, and messing with their daily function.

Now, we all know the obvious: proper diet; adequate exercise;

plenty of water; sufficient sleep. In fact So far, physical activity and weight loss appear to be the key. Several new studies indicate that regular exercise, such as brisk walking for 30 to 45 minutes a day, can significantly decrease such fat.

At greatest risk of developing health problems from too much hidden belly fat are men whose waists are wider than 40 inches and women whose waists are wider than 35 inches.

But, there are a couple of nutritional supplements that may be of interest. One is CLA (conjugated linoleic acid). While CLA has been known since the 1930's, the real benefits of CLA started to be explored in 1987. CLA (conjugated linoleic acid) has been shown to be very effective in reducing waist size. The weight around your waist is fat. CLA helps burn and liberate fat–so it can have great results around your middle. This is contrast to many diet pills that really just help you lose water weight. Clinical studies have shown CLA to be effective in reducing body fat and increasing lean muscle mass. The most recent 1 year human study, in the American Journal of Clinical Nutrition, showed a reduction in body fat and increase in muscle mass. Contrary to early reports, CLA does NOT appear to be a useful supplement for people with diabetes, and might in fact contribute to diabetes in overweight people. In addition, it might increase cardiovascular risk in another manner.

The typical dosage of CLA ranges from 3000- 5000 mg daily. As with all supplements taken at this high a dosage, it is important to purchase a reputable brand, as even very small amounts of toxic contaminants in any medication or supplement could quickly add up.

Chromium is an essential trace mineral for the human body. Chromium supplements are often sold for weight loss, particularly for obese people who may be in danger of developing diabetes. Scientists have been studying the supplement's potential role in weight control. The best and safest source of chromium is food. Whole grains, ready-to-eat bran cereals, seafood, green beans, broccoli, prunes, nuts, peanut butter, and potatoes are rich in chromium. Sugary foods are low in this mineral and may even promote chromium loss; vitamin C may increase its absorption. Don't exceed the amount in multivitamin/mineral pills—20 to 120 micrograms—that preferably should not be in the form of chromium picolinate.

GUM DISEASE
AND YOUR HEALTH

⸻

Oral Health is important to overall health and general well-being; you cannot be healthy without oral health. There is little doubt that oral health and general well-being are closely linked. Almost 3 of every 10 adults over age 65 have lost all of their teeth, primarily because of tooth decay and gum disease, which affects about 25% of U.S. adults. Tooth loss has more than cosmetic effects—it may contribute to nutrition problems by limiting the types of food that a person can eat.

Just as routine medical exams can help prevent future health problems, and dental exams are equally important. The evidence shows that an infection from periodontitis, or gum disease, can put you at risk for other serious conditions like heart disease, stroke and more!

What you may not realize is that oral health is not just important for maintaining a nice-looking smile and being able to eat corn on the cob. Good oral health is essential to quality of life. Consider a few of the reasons:

- Every tooth in your mouth plays an important role in speaking, chewing and in maintaining proper alignment of other teeth.
- A major cause of failure in joint replacements is infection, which can travel to the site of the replacement from the mouth in people with periodontal disease.
- People with dentures or loose and missing teeth often have restricted diets since biting into fresh fruits and vegetables are often not only difficult, but also painful. This likely means they don't get proper nutrition.
- Most men and women age 65 and older report that a smile is very important to a person's appearance.
- And, maybe most importantly, recent research has advanced the idea that periodontal disease is linked to a number of major health concerns such as heart disease, stroke, respiratory disease and diabetes.

Fifty percent of all people over the age of 18 have at least the early stage of gum disease, gingivitis. Gum disease at one time or another afflicts Three out of four over the age of 35.

You should be aware that the early stages of gum disease occurs WITHOUT PAIN! Yet, your gums and bones may be silently and seriously damaged by an infection that spreads from your gums to other parts of your body! Also, perfectly healthy teeth can eventually become loose and fall out.

More than half of older patients do not understand taking certain medications may affect the health of their mouth. For example, many medications, including diuretics, may reduce salivary flow. Dry mouth can cause increased plaque buildup, which increases the risk for periodontal disease. In addition, some calcium channel blockers may cause the gums to grow over the teeth.

Dental Infections Do Go BEYOND Your Gums:

- **Stroke:** A new study of fatty deposits lodged in the carotid arteries of stroke sufferer's shows that 70% contain bacteria—and 40% of those bacteria come from the mouth.

- **Heart Disease:** Bacteria get mixed up with blood-clotting cells called platelets, forming a clump that travels through the blood vessel and may promote the formation of heart-stopping blood clots.

- **Lungs:** It has been shown that those with extensive tartar build-up and plaque on their teeth are at risk for chronic lung disease, including chronic obstructive pulmonary disease and pneumonia.

- **Diabetes:** One study showed that diabetics with gum disease were three times more likely to have heart attacks than those without gum disease.

- **Spontaneous Pre-Term Births (for women):** Women with gum disease are 7 to 8 times more likely to give birth prematurely to low-birth-weight babies. Researchers believe that a low-grade infection, often from gum disease, may be linked to pre-term birth.

Women who are menopausal or post-menopausal may experience changes in their mouths. Recent studies suggest that estrogen deficiency could place post-menopausal women at higher risk for severe peri-odontal disease and tooth loss.

In addition, hormonal changes in older women may result in discomfort in the mouth, including dry mouth, pain and burning sensations in the gum tissue and altered taste, especially salty, pep-pery or sour.

Bone loss is associated with both periodontal disease and osteopo-rosis. Osteoporosis could lead to tooth loss because the density of the bone that supports the teeth may be decreased. More research is being done to determine if and how a relationship between osteoporosis and periodontal disease exists.

To keep your teeth for a lifetime, you must remove the plaque from your teeth and gums every day with proper brushing and flossing. Regular dental visits are also important. Daily cleaning will help keep calculus formation to a minimum, but it won't completely prevent it. A professional cleaning at least twice a year is necessary to remove calcu-lus from places your toothbrush and floss may have missed.

The good news is that gum disease is easy to prevent by maintain-ing basic oral health steps.

See a periodontist if you or your dentist notices problems with your gum tissue. Problems may include:

- Bleeding gums during brushing
- Red, swollen or tender gums
- Gums that have pulled away from the teeth
- Persistent bad breath
- Pus between the teeth and gums

Gum Disease and Your Health

- Loose or separating teeth
- A change in the way your teeth fit together when you bite
- A change in the fit of your dentures

Oral health is often taken for granted, but it is an essential part of our everyday lives. Good oral health enhances our ability to speak, smile, smell, taste, touch, chew, swallow, and convey our feelings and emotions through facial expressions. However, oral diseases, which range from cavities to oral cancer, cause pain and disability.

The effect that gum disease has on overall health is directly related to the extent and duration of the infection. Moderate to advanced gum disease exposes the body to excessive amounts of harmful bacteria 24 hours a day, seven days a week, for as long as the infection is present. The stress this bacterial infection can place on the immune system is significant and it can dramatically reduce the body's ability to fight other infections and diseases.

While the nation's politicians are battling like kids, we should not overlook the role dental health plays in the cost of health care in this country.

Many studies have provided evidence of the dramatic effect of gum disease on health care costs. In 2007, in the US alone, we spent $2.2 TRILLION on health care. One study demonstrated that 21% of total health care costs could be saved by eliminating gum disease. That is nearly $500 billion dollars a year in savings simply by eliminating gum disease.

USE CAUTION WITH
NATURAL MEDICINE

═══════════════

For years, I have been filled with anxiety, as I watched explosion of the "cottage industry" of herbalists; naturopaths; "holistic" doctors, and the like. Now, some of will quickly point out that I, too, was once mostly known for my contribution to this growing population. But, like any good sinner, I have repented, and vowed to sin no more. (Thank you, Dr. Edward S. Cooper!)

Let me explain. Over thirty years ago, after being a Pre-Med student, I made a decision not to go on to medical school, and instead direct my interests and talents to supporting the ability of people to take better control of their own lives and their health. This led me down a long path (that included years of working with Dick Gregory), and ultimately to being, what some consider an important voice in health advocacy and health education.

Included in my journey were "stops" as an herbalist; homeopath' health store owner; health columnist and lecturer; and a media commentator.

Use Caution with Natural Medicine

The most disturbing part of these experiences, as a "sinner", was the speed at which people were prepared to do, or take, whatever I suggested for them to take to "cure what ails them". Never mind that they were under the care of a medical doctor for serious medical conditions.

The resulting effect on me was to do two things: 1) do everything I can to make sure that anything I said or wrote was based on as much scientific and/or researched information as possible. I read and study as much as any medical doctor or scientist. 2) I strongly adhere to the premise that there is no "alternative" to a medical doctor. This has led me to be a strong proponent of Complementary and Alternative Medicine (CAM). What it means is that I don't do, say, or suggest anything to anyone without the knowledge and/or approval of their medical doctor.

I shudder when I hear of people who brag about ignoring their doctors' recommendations because either "they don't believe in Doctors' medicine", or because "an herbalist looked into their eyes" and said that they had just the thing for their medical condition.

I recently heard a story about a tragic example of how wrong these types of decisions can go, and how costly (in terms of life and permanent risk to health).

For years, I have not written or spoke publicly on my disdain for what I consider to be charlatan (somebody who falsely claims to have special skill or expertise) behavior in the name of "healing' people, and helping them learn the "natural way". But as these incidents continue to happen more and more, and families are devastated by the senseless loss or injury of a loved one, I am silent no more. I have to live with my own conscience. I have been given the privilege of being a source of trusted and valued information, and so add this to the growing list of topics I will write about.

Information is the Best Medicine

The use of dietary supplements has risen tremendously in recent years. Increasingly, people now take herbs and other "natural" substances in addition to vitamins and minerals. These so-called nutritional products are not as strictly regulated under the law as prescription drugs, however, and to use them wisely, consumers should know about the risks and benefits associated with supplements. Dietary supplements are billed as immune triggers, weight-loss wonders, "brain power", muscle-expanding elixirs, and much more. They can be bought from the shelves of health food stores, drug stores, and supermarkets. They are a category of nutritional additives that once included just vitamins and minerals, but now also encompass herbs, amino acids, fish oils, hormones, and many other substances. Not only is the array of supplements dazzling, but also their popularity is soaring.

Sales of vitamins and minerals in America alone have reached $25 billion annually! And with the USA accounting for barely 5% of the world's population, we buy over 30% of all of these supplements. The reason for this is partly as a result of rising medical costs which encourages both prevention and self-care. Like many things, African Americans, and other underserved communities, are impacted disproportionately, and turn to these "alternatives" in larger relative numbers.

Even science has lent credibility to a handful of the claims made for dietary supplements. Some studies have suggested, for example, that vitamins may help prevent serious illnesses such as heart disease and cancer. All this has fed a media frenzy regarding the latest research into natural remedies. We see Madison Avenue using people, places and things we care about to appeal to our emotions, just as would in selling us cars and "happy meals". I was shocked (even though I shouldn't have been) to hear a prominent national civil rights leader as a spokesperson for a "new" herbal product for men's prostate conditions.

At the same time, supplements of all kinds have moved from niche retailers such as health food stores into drugstores and supermarkets, making them more widely available and also more appealing to the mainstream public. And the claims have gone far beyond what science has shown, appealing to everybody from athletes to people with chronic diseases.

"True" herbalism encompasses scientific testing, honest reporting of the results, and safe use of effective herbs by informed practitioners and the public. It also includes the production and ethical marketing of herbal products. True herbalism, which brings honor to the wonder-filled world of plants, <u>does</u> exist as part of the science of pharmacology. However, there is a dark side to herbalism.

Herbal medicine has long been an alternative for those seeking health-related remedies without using powerful pharmaceuticals. While these herbs tend to have a lesser degree of side effects, they can still cause adverse reactions if used improperly.

Herbal medicines, like other forms of medications, can sometimes contain other additives to help preserve the pill or enhance the effect of the herb. It is important to be aware of what is in your herbal medicines, particularly if you are allergic to certain additives. This information is sometimes readily available on the bottle; at other times, you may have to do some research before beginning to ingest any herb.

For the many untested pills, capsules, powders, and liquids that remain on the shelves, it pays to be cautious. Here are a few tips for dealing with the supplement conundrum:

- Before taking a supplement, find out what evidence supports its advertised benefits-and dangers.
- It is a good idea to glean information from a variety of sources, not just one book or magazine article.
- Learn what "real" scientists know about safe dosages and do not exceed them.

Somewhere, as you read this column, there is someone either dead or suffering from not having the benefit of this information.

Everyone knows consumers buy supplements to prevent or treat what ails them in order to escape the sometimes adverse, allergic, or dizzying side effects they've had from prescription drugs. The reason people buy supplements is to have a better quality of life. Consumers also want a safer quality of supplements and foods. People buy supplements also out of fear.

The real questions are not whether the supplements make you healthier, but are they safe? Are you sure that the person "prescribing" seems to know what they're talking about, but are they really trained in helping you or are you just a good customer? How do these people become "Doctors" anyway?

HOW MEDICINES CAN AFFECT THE DIGESTIVE SYSTEM

Many medicines taken by mouth may affect the digestive system. These medicines include prescription (those ordered by a doctor and dispensed by a pharmacist) and nonprescription or over-the-counter (OTC) products. Although these medicines usually are safe and effective, harmful effects may occur in some people.

In fact many people not only suffer, but also start taking another medicine to address the problems caused by taking a normally prescribed medication properly.

Here are some of the ways in which prescription medicines can affect you:

THE ESOPHAGUS

Some people have difficulty swallowing medicines in tablet or capsule

131

form. Tablets or capsules that stay in the esophagus may release chemicals that irritate the lining of the esophagus. The irritation may cause ulcers, bleeding, perforation (a hole or tear), and strictures (narrowing) of the esophagus. The risk of pill-induced injuries to the esophagus increases in persons with conditions involving the esophagus, such as strictures, scleroderma (hardening of the skin), achalasia (irregular muscle activity of the esophagus, which delays the passage of food), and stroke.

Some medicines can cause ulcers when they become lodged in the esophagus. These medicines include aspirin, several antibiotics such as tetracycline, potassium chloride, vitamin C, and iron.

ESOPHAGEAL REFLUX

The lower esophageal sphincter (LES) muscle is between the esophagus and the stomach. The muscle allows the passage of food into the stomach after swallowing, and then prevents passage back into the esophagus. Certain medicines interfere with the action of the sphincter muscle, which increases the likelihood of backup or reflux of the highly acidic contents of the stomach into the esophagus.

Medicines that can cause esophageal reflux include nitrates, diuretics, calcium channel blockers, and birth control pills.

THE STOMACH

One of the most common drug-induced injuries is irritation of the lining of the stomach caused by non-steroidal anti-inflammatory drugs (NSAIDs).

NSAIDs can irritate the stomach by weakening the ability of the lining to resist acid made in the stomach. Sometimes this irritation may lead to inflammation of the stomach lining (gastritis), ulcers, bleeding, or perforation of the lining. Older people are especially at risk for irritation from NSAIDs because they are more likely to regularly take pain medicines for arthritis and other chronic conditions. Also at risk are folks with a history of peptic ulcers and related complications or gastritis.

DELAYED EMPTYING OF THE STOMACH

Some medicines cause nerve and muscle activity to slow down in the stomach. This slowing down causes the contents of the stomach to empty at a slower rate than normal.

Drugs that may cause this delay include drugs used to treat Parkinson's disease and depression.

CONSTIPATION

Constipation can be caused by a variety of medicines. These medicines affect the nerve and muscle activity in the large intestine (colon). This results in the slow and difficult passage of stool. Medicines also may bind intestinal liquid and make the stool hard.

Medicines that commonly cause constipation include high blood pressure drugs, anxiety drugs, cholesterol drugs, iron, and antacids that contain mostly aluminum.

DIARRHEA

Diarrhea is a common side effect of many medicines. Diarrhea is often caused by antibiotics, which affect the bacteria that live normally in the large intestine.

Antibiotic-induced changes in intestinal bacteria allow overgrowth of other bacteria, which is the cause of a more serious antibiotic-induced diarrhea.

Diarrhea also can be a side effect of drugs that alter the movements or fluid content of the colon. Magnesium-containing antacids can have the effect of laxatives and cause diarrhea if overused. In addition, the abuse of laxatives may result in damage to the nerves and muscles of the colon and cause diarrhea.

The Liver

The liver processes most medicines that enter the bloodstream and governs drug activity throughout the body. Once a drug enters the bloodstream, the liver converts the drug into chemicals the body can use and removes toxic chemicals that other organs cannot tolerate. During this process, these chemicals can attack and injure the liver.

Drug-induced liver injury can resemble the symptoms of any acute or chronic liver disease. The only way a doctor can diagnose drug-induced liver injury is by stopping use of the suspected drug and excluding other liver diseases through diagnostic tests. Rarely, long-term use of a medicine can cause chronic liver damage and scarring (cirrhosis).

Medicines that can cause severe liver injury include large doses of acetaminophen (and even in small doses when taken with alcohol), and vitamins such as vitamin A and niacin.

Always talk with your doctor before taking a medicine (prescription and OTC's) for the first time and before adding any new medicines to those you already are taking. Certain medicines taken together may interact and cause harmful side effects. In addition, tell your doctor about any allergies or sensitivities to foods and medicines and about any medical conditions you may have such as diabetes, kidney disease, or liver disease.

Be sure that you understand all directions for taking the medicine, including dose and schedule, possible interactions with food, alcohol, and other medicines, side effects, and warnings. If you are an older adult, read all directions carefully and ask your doctor questions about the medicine. As you get older, you may be more susceptible to drug interactions that cause side effects.

As you get older you may be faced with more health conditions that you need to treat on a regular basis. It is important to be aware that more use of medicines and normal body changes caused by aging can increase the chance of unwanted or maybe even harmful drug interactions. As you age, body changes can affect the way medicines are absorbed and used. For example, changes in the digestive system can affect how fast medicines enter the bloodstream. Changes in body weight can influence the amount of medicine you need to take and how long it stays in your body. The circulation system may slow down, which can affect how fast drugs get to the liver and kidneys. The liver and kidneys also may work more slowly affecting the way a drug breaks down and is removed from the body. Because of these body changes, there is also a bigger risk of drug interactions for older adults. Drug-drug interactions happen when two or more medicines react with each other to cause unwanted effects. This kind of interaction can also cause one medicine to not work as well or even make one medicine stronger than it should be. For example, you should not take aspirin if you are taking a prescription blood thinner, such as Warfarin, unless your health care professional tells you to.

INFORMATION IS THE BEST MEDICINE

The more you know about your medicines and the more you talk with your health care professionals, the easier it is to avoid problems with medicines–especially in your digestive system.

INFO ON ACID REFLUX

Do you suffer from heartburn? Does it seem like no matter what you eat, heartburn keeps occurring?

Gastroesophageal reflux disease, commonly referred to as GERD or acid reflux, is a condition in which the liquid content of the stomach regurgitates (backs up or refluxes) into the esophagus. GERD is a chronic condition. Once it begins, it usually is life-long.

The stomach's first job is to accept and store the food that enters it. In response to the arrival of food, glands present in the lining of the stomach produce stomach acid (or gastric acid)–another digestive juice.

Muscles in the wall of the stomach help to move the food and acid around making sure that they mix thoroughly. Stomach acid helps to break down the food further into smaller, easier to digest fragments.

Some of the benefits of a good acid supply are:

- needed for proper calcium absorption
- kills bacteria and viruses etc.
- facilitates proper digestion of protein

What nature intended is that you eat enzyme rich foods and chew your food properly. If you did that, the food would enter the stomach laced with digestive enzymes. These enzymes would then "predigest" your food for about an hour — actually breaking down as much as 75% of your meal.

Only after this period of "pre-digestion" are hydrochloric acid and pepsin introduced. Once this concentrate enters the small intestine, the acid is neutralized and the pancreas reintroduces digestive enzymes to the process. As digestion is completed, nutrients are passed through the intestinal wall and into the bloodstream.

That's what nature intended. Unfortunately, most of us don't live our lives as nature intended!

Processing and cooking destroy enzymes in food. (Any sustained heat of approximately 118–129 F destroys virtually all enzymes.) This means that, for most of us, the food entering our stomach is severely enzyme deficient. The food then sits there for an hour, like a heavy lump, with very little pre-digestion taking place. This forces the body to produce large amounts of stomach acid in an attempt to overcompensate.

A lot of people try drinking milk to ease acid reflux before sleep. But often, milk ends up causing acid reflux during sleep. To understand the whole situation, we have to realize that the problem roots from eating too much at dinnertime. Eating a big meal at dinner causes excess stomach acid production. Drinking milk could be a quick fix to the acid reflux problem. Unfortunately, milk has a rebound action and would eventually encourage secretion of more stomach acid, which causes the acid reflux. To solve the problem, try adjusting your diet by eating a small meal at dinner and have a small snack such as crackers before sleep.

Info on Acid Reflux

First of all, try to eat small, frequent meals instead of three big meals a day. Small amounts of food each time would exert less workload on the stomach and therefore requires less acid secretion for digestion. Make sure to include foods that are high in complex __carbohydrates__ in each meal. These foods, such as rice, breads and pasta, are able to tie up excess stomach acid and are often easy on the stomach.

High fat foods will remain in the stomach longer, thus causing the need for more stomach acid in order to digest them. Be sure to avoid or limit alcohol. The worst of all is beer. It could double your stomach acid within an hour.

Over a long period of time chronic acid reflux wears away the lower esophageal sphincter or LES, which is the valve which keeps stomach acid and its contents in the stomach, and mechanically prevents a normal amount of stomach acid from washing into the esophagus, and upper throat. When the LES becomes damaged beyond a certain degree from acid reflux, it is no longer capable of performing its function, and acid reflux will be experienced unless surgery is performed to repair the damage.

When refluxed stomach acid touches the lining of the esophagus, it causes a burning sensation in the chest or throat called heartburn. The fluid may even be tasted in the back of the mouth, and this is called acid indigestion. Occasional heartburn is common but does not necessarily mean one has chronic acid reflux disease. Heartburn that occurs more than twice a week may be considered "Chronic Acid Reflux Disease", and it can eventually lead to more serious health problems.

Depending on how severe your "Chronic Acid Reflux is, treatment may involve one or more of the following lifestyle changes and medications or surgery.

Supplementing with digestive enzymes to reduce the need for stomach acid — giving the body a chance to rest and recover its ability to produce sufficient stomach acid.

Mix one teaspoon of apple cider vinegar with water and a little honey and drink this with each meal. You may gradually increase the vinegar up to 3-4 tablespoons in water if needed.

Supplementing with betaine hydrochloride (HCL) tablets can also help, but anything beyond minimal doses as found in most health food store supplements should only be administered under the supervision of a health practitioner to avoid damage to the stomach lining.

When you experience chronic heartburn, the first step to controlling your heartburn is to record what may trigger your attacks, the severity of the attacks, how your body reacts, and what gives you relief. The next step is to take this information to your doctor so the both of you can determine what lifestyle changes you will need to make and what treatments will give you maximum relief.

If you have been using antacids for more than 2 weeks, it is time to see a doctor.

BOWEL MOVEMENTS: SINKERS OR FLOATERS?

B y popular demand, here is a re-visit to a topic that few dare to explore – bowel movements.

A regular bowel movement is normally considered essential for good general health. But in most cases less frequent bowel movements are common and not necessarily a cause for concern. How to have a regular bowel movement and bowel or defecation habits vary from person to person.

Your bowel movement can tell you a lot about your health. This may not be a topic you would typically talked about at the dinner table or a party, but actually more people are somewhat obsessed with it than you would imagine. We should be interested the appearance and/or condition of our bowel movement.

The general health or state of your gastro-intestinal tract or GI tract and the quality and quantity of its output is a great indicator of the health of your body. The GI tract is a rather high tech processing unit. It metabolizes all of the nutrients you take in and eliminates all of the body's waste that is generated. What comes through it, the bowel movement or stool is insightful of how well or how ill the body is.

There are certain medications, such as blood pressure drugs, antidepressants and anti histamines—that can slow down the GI tract. Constipation or irregular bowel movements, which has a myriad of causes, will lead to even harder, drier stools (since you're going less often, your stool will stall in the system and the fluid is re-absorbed. For some people, consuming a diet high in dairy products can be a cause of constipation. So, if you are experiencing problems going and have dry, hard-to-pass stool when you do finally go, try reducing your dairy intake for a week or two to see if that helps. Then again, being dehydrated can also lead to this problem. If the body is lacking in water, your system will draw it, and conserve it, from wherever it can find it.

The quality of your bowel movements is nature's way of telling you the level of health you are experiencing. Just as you need to monitor what goes in your mouth, stool investigation will give you valuable information regarding your highway to health, the digestive tract.

There is a reason for the large intestine to be the first organ developed in the fetus. It is the most important and influential organ of the body. Without proper sanitation, life cannot exist. The best signs that your sewer system is not functioning properly are: bad breath, smelly stools, and there's no way you can leave the bathroom without the use of air freshener!

What indicates a good bowel movement is, firstly, that the stool floats. Floating stools are both a blessing and a curse. They can float because they are so full of bubbles and gas that they are abnormal. On the other hand, they float because they have too much fat in them, or they can float because they are high in fiber, which is the kind we want.

Now, here's the big question:

Do you produce floaters or sinkers when you have a bowel movement?

It is not the weight of your stools, but rather their densities that determines their out-of-body fate to *float or to sink*. Simply put, the "floaters" are bloated by the air in them. Sinkers need a lot more fiber in their diet.

Floaters may be caused by gas in the stool, resulting from a change in the diet. Perhaps you've suddenly started eating more high fiber foods, for example. Undigested fat will also make stools float. This could be an indication that your diet is too high in fat, or there could be a problem with nutrient absorption in your diet. Stools that result from poor food absorption often leave a greasy film on the water and are rather large.

If you're suffering from constipation, you may produce impacted stools, which will "sink" because of their density and lack of moisture. You need to include more fiber, both soluble and insoluble, in your diet to bulk out the stools and get your digestive system working properly again. And drink more water. The bowel and colon need water to work efficiently, just like the rest of your body.

The truth is, a healthy stool is neither a sinker nor a floater–it's a combination of the two. If you're in good general health, you'll pass some sinkers, some floaters and some that seem to just sit in the water, neither floating nor sinking. As long as your bowel motions are soft, fairly bulky and easy and painless to pass, and there's no sign of blood or excessive mucus in the stools, everything is well down below.

We want stools that do not mark the toilet bowel. We want them to hang together and not be pebbles, non-stinking, have no undigested food particles, a large volume, a clean wiping, and a definite sense of complete evacuation.

Wiping clean should only take a few pieces of toilet paper – not a roll. It is amazing how often people do NOT have this sense of complete evacuation. We want one or more bowel movements every day.

The digestive process can vary depending on what is being eaten and the person's metabolism. For example, fat takes alot longer to digest than sugars. Fiber in the diet speeds up transit time (the amount of time from chewing to bowel movement). Generally it can range from 24 to 48 hours for men and slightly longer for women. Chewing takes 5 to 30 seconds followed by swallowing for up to 10 seconds. The food enters the stomach where it is churned and broken apart by harsh acids, namely hydrochloric acid. The food can remain in the stomach from 1 to 4 hours after which it empties in a semi liquid form called chyme into the small intestine. Here is where most of the real digestion takes place.

In other words most of the nutrients are absorbed from the small intestine into the blood stream. The highly acidic nature of the chyme is neutralized by the pancreas with bicarbonates and bile from the gallbladder and liver. This process can take about 3 to 6 hours. Finally about 10 hours after you've eaten the mushy paste of undigested food enters the large intestine or colon. Here it may take another 18 hours or even up to 2 days before its elimination as feces. Water and certain vitamins are absorbed from the colon but most of the waste consists of indigestible bits of food, mostly fibers from fruit, vegetables and grains.

The amount of time (intestinal transit time) it takes for the food you eat to make its way through the gastro-intestinal system and then exit into the toilet will have an impact on the consistency of your stool. Intestinal transit can vary greatly. It depends on your general health and diet. For a person in generally good health and eating a healthy diet, the intestinal transit time will be about 12–24 hours. The average American will have a transit time of 40 to 45 hours. The longer the waste or stool stays in the GI tract, the more fluid is re-absorbed into the body and the stool becomes harder and dryer.

So you see transit time for a meal can vary anywhere from 22 hours up to two days.

And there you have it, "from the tooter to the rooter"!

THE TRUTH ABOUT CARBS

What's all the fuss about carbs? Low carb foods, no carb diets. Just what is carbohydrate? Should you avoid it because it makes you fat?

There is little doubt that the human body uses carbohydrates most efficiently for energy production (as opposed to fats and proteins). So there isn't really any reason to avoid carbs, even if you're trying to lose weight. But there is a BIG difference between the natural, wholesome, 'good' carbs we are designed to eat and the unnatural, highly-processed, 'refined' carbs so many of us consume on a daily basis!

These 'bad' carbs are contributing to a health crisis in America and other parts of the world in the forms of obesity, diabetes, heart disease, and cancer. Millions of people are simply unaware of what they are doing to their bodies every time they eat processed carbs. What's worse, many parents don't realize that they are setting their kids up for a lifetime of health problems by allowing them to develop the 'junk food habit' at a young age.

Bad carbs are refined, processed carbohydrate foods that have had all or most of their natural nutrients and fiber removed in order to make them easier to transport and more 'consumer friendly.' Most baked goods, white breads, pastas, snack foods, candies, and non-diet soft drinks fit into this category. Bleached, enriched wheat flour and white sugar–along with an array of artificial flavorings, colorings, and preservatives–are the most common ingredients used to make 'bad carb' foods.

Bad carbs are harmful mainly because the human body is not able to process them very well. Our hormonal and digestive systems developed over the course of millions of years. Yet only in the past 100 years or so have humans had access to these highly processed carbohydrates in abundance. Our bodies simply didn't have time to adapt and evolve to handle the rapid changes in food processing.

Because of this, most of the processed carbs we eat wreak havoc on our natural hormone levels. Insulin production, especially, is 'thrown out of wack' as the body attempts to process the huge amounts of starches and simple sugars contained in a typical 'bad carb'-based meal. This leads to dramatic fluctuations in blood glucose levels–a big reason why you often feel lethargic after eating these unhealthy meals.

Also, it's important to realize that most processed carb foods provide only 'empty' calories–calories with little or no nutritional-value. Eat enough of these empty calories and your body will quickly turn them into extra body fat, as anyone with a weight problem already knows all to well!

The regular consumption of large amounts of high-sugar, low-fiber, nutritionally-poor 'bad carbs' eventually leads to a much higher risk of obesity, diabetes, cancer, heart disease, and more. It's pretty clear that the abundance of processed carbs and unhealthy trans-fats found in so many foods is a major cause–if not the biggest cause–of many of our modern chronic health problems.

Carbohydrates provide energy for the body. Once consumed, they travel to the liver, which breaks them down into glucose, or blood sugar. Carbohydrates are especially used to provide energy to the brain and to the central nervous system. Carbohydrates are labeled as complex or simple. This reflects how fast the sugar is absorbed into the bloodstream.

Eating too many foods high in carbohydrates can cause your calorie intake to go up, making you gain unwanted weight. Alternately, a lack of carbohydrates can cause malnutrition and weaknesses. Carbohydrates provide most of the energy the body needs to function. About 55% of your energy foods should come from different varieties of carbohydrates. Much more than that, however, can be detrimental to health. Someone who derives 75% or more of total energy from carbohydrates can be lacking in protein and fats.

Health problem can develop when someone eats too many complex carbohydrates that contain refined sugars. These sugars lack vitamins and fiber but offer a lot of calories. Eating too much refined sugar will lead to weight gain. Examples of these foods include white flour, polished rice, table sugar, and white pasta. A good rule to remember when eating carbohydrates is to eat them in as natural a form as possible.

Here are five basic guidelines for carbohydrate consumption that are based on current scientific knowledge:

- *Get most of your carbs from fruits and vegetables.* Carbohydrate is the primary macronutrient in fruits and vegetables. In other words, these foods contain a lot more carbohydrate than protein or fat.

- *Eat whole grains instead of processed grains whenever possible.* There's nothing wrong with including a moderate amount of grains (wheat, rice, etc.) in your diet, but these grains should be whole grains such as brown rice rather than refined grains such as white flour. Refined grains have been stripped of their fiber, a type of indigestible carbohydrate that slows the absorption of other carbohydrates, and most of their other nutrients.

- *Vary your carb intake with your activity level.* Unlike protein and fat, carbs are used only to provide immediate energy for mental and physical activity. Any carbs consumed in excess of the amount needed to meet immediate physical and mental energy needs are converted to body fat. So the amount of carbohydrate you consume needs to be determined by your activity level. If you don't exercise and have an office job, you should not consume more than three or four grams of carbohydrate per pound of body weight daily. If you perform physical work or exercise moderately, aim for five or six grams per pound. If you are highly active, seven or eight grams of carbohydrate per pound of body weight will be needed to keep your body functioning optimally.

- *Strictly limit your sugar intake.* The sugars that are added to foods such as cookies and candy bars and to beverages such as lattes and energy drinks should be avoided as much as possible. They add a lot of calories to these products and thereby promote weight gain. Consuming large amounts of sugar over many years may also increase the risk of type 2 diabetes independently of weight gain. If there truly is any "bad carb," sugar is it.

- *Pay attention to how carbs affect you physically and mentally.* Different people react to carbohydrates differently. Some people absorb carbs in foods much faster than others do and are thus more susceptible to "blood sugar crashes" an hour or two after eating a high-carbohydrate meal. Pay attention to how you feel and function after consuming large amounts of carbs and adjust your diet accordingly. If you feel lethargic and perform poorly after eating carbs, you should reduce the amount of carbohydrate in your diet.

- *Eat protein with your carbs.* When protein is consumed with carbohydrate, the carbs are absorbed more slowly and the meal is more filling. It's a good idea to consume some form of lean protein whenever you consume carbohydrate-rich foods.

You can't talk about carbs without mentioning the glycemic index (GI). The GI is a way of comparing different carbs by ranking their effect on blood sugar levels.

The glycemic index of food is a ranking of foods based on their immediate effect on blood glucose (blood sugar) levels. Carbohydrate foods that breakdown quickly during digestion have the highest glycemic indexes. Their blood sugar response is fast and high. Carbohydrates that breakdown slowly, releasing glucose gradually into the blood stream, have low glycemic indexes. What is the significance of Glycemic Index?

- Low GI means a smaller rise in blood sugar and can help control established diabetes
- Low GI diets can help people lose weight and lower blood lipids
- Low GI diets can improve the body's sensitivity to insulin
- High GI foods can help re-fuel carbohydrate stores after exercise

How to switch to a low GI diet

- Breakfast cereals based on wheat bran, barley and oats
- "Grainy" breads made with whole seeds
- Pasta and rice in place of potatoes
- Vinegar and lemon juice dressings

In short, the goal should be to build a good plan including the low Glycemic Index foods. This way, hunger is minimized, and there is less of a tendency to "cheat" or overeat. Consequently, you can continue to lose body fat or maintain your weight–once the excess pounds have been lost. Even for those whose main objective is not fat loss, foods that are low on the glycemic index will help alleviate mood swings and regulate energy levels.

DIFFICULTY IN
LOSING WEIGHT

===

As we approach the end of every year, most of us are focused on another opportunity to resume our "battle of the bulge". Yes, the New Year brings with it renewed promised to get the weight loss thing right, once and for all.

Let me share a recent experience with one of my readers, which might make it easier for you to claim victory this time around.

A few days ago, a man who I was consulting in his treatment strategy to treat prostate cancer, called me after his most recent visit to his doctor. He was noticeably shaken, after being told that as serious as his prostate cancer was, the greatest threat to his health was his obesity. In fact, the told him he was morbidly obese.

Now, this guy was baffled. After all, he thought, since he was diagnosed with prostate cancer, he had drastically changed his diet. Yet he had actually gained three (3) pounds.

I did my best to calm him, reassure him, and encouraged him to keep on this newly modified diet and lifestyle.

I am finding there are many men who find themselves in the same situation- making a strong determination to lose weight, but to no avail!

Here are some possible reasons why:

1. You could actually be Starving!

Slashing too many calories, particularly protein calories, pushes the body to conserve calories rather than burn them. It also forces your body to break down muscle tissue to fuel its vital operations. But that muscle is the key to your metabolism, or the speed at which you burn calories. More muscle means a faster metabolism and less body fat.

Solution: You do need to cut calories to lose weight. (Cut 500 today by eliminating one can of beer, 30 chips, and one Oreo from your diet.) But you need to make sure you're eating at least 1,600 to 1,800 calories each day to keep your metabolism from shutting down. And never cut protein during a diet. If you're a sedentary 200-pounder, you need about 75 grams of protein (about two chicken breasts) a day for muscle preservation. If you're lifting weights, aim for twice that much. Doing aerobics? Pick a number in between.

2. You're "Inhaling" Food

You probably eat so fast that your stomach hardly has time to alert your brain to tell your mouth to quit chewing before your stomach explodes.

Solution: On every bite, chew, swallow, put down your fork, and take a sip of water. See how long it takes you to eat.

3. YOUR FOOD IS TOO REFINED

Most processed breads and cereals contain little fiber, the calorie-free component of plant foods that fills you up, not out. Plus, foods rich in fiber help control blood glucose and insulin levels.

Solution: I never thought I'd say this, but it may be a good idea to cut back on potatoes in any form (especially the fries, fellas). Experts say potatoes raise blood-glucose concentration quickly, as do snack chips, white bread, low-fiber breakfast cereals, and breakfast bars. Whole-grain cereals, nuts, and beans are blame-free, if not calorie-free.

4. YOU ARE TIRED

Sleep deprivation decreases the odds of shedding blubber and keeping it off. Researchers found that healthy men who snoozed only 4 or 7 hours a night for 6 nights in a row had higher glucose and insulin levels in their blood. This is a terrible state of metabolism for a man who's trying to lose weight, because surplus insulin boosts body-fat storage.

Solution: Hit the sack for 8 hours each and every night. And try to hit it for the same 8 hours.

5. YOU THINK FITNESS "OUTWEIGHS" FATNESS

Exercise alone won't make you thin. A recent study of military personnel who increased their exercise during a 3-year period found that they gained weight despite their extra efforts. Why? Food, most likely. They simply ate more than they burned off.

Solution: Controlling portion size is absolutely essential to weight loss. And the best way to control portion size is to limit how often you eat out. According to the Tufts University Health & Nutrition Letter, a single restaurant meal often could feed an entire family

6. YOU LACK BASIC FOOD-PREPARATIONS SKILLS

A man whose only kitchen skill involves the speed dial to Domino's is condemned to a diet of grease, salt, white bread, and sugar.

Solution: Step into the kitchen. (That's the room with the oven, sink, and refrigerator.) Open your freezer. You should see frozen berries and vegetables, which are as good as fresh but last many times longer. Look in your cupboards. You should see some canned vegetables, hearty low-fat soups, dried fruit, and slow-cooking oats. These foods help you lose weight because they're filling but low in calories

7. YOU'RE DRY

When you're trying to lose weight, water is your workout partner. You need it to flush the waste products your body makes when it breaks down fat for energy, or when it processes protein. You need it to transport nutrients to your muscles. You need it to help digest food and keep your metabolism clicking along. And water keeps you from overheating during intense exercise on hot days.

8. MACHO MACHO MAN

I've seen it many times: Guy drops 10 or 20 pounds and starts thinking he's Joe Weight Loss. Next thing you know, he's back to beer and pizza—and his original weight.

Solution: With each 10 pounds you drop, sit down and reassess your diet and exercise program. If you calculated your food intake and exercise volume when you started, run a new set of numbers, based on your new weight and activity level.

These are just a few observations, but I'm sure you'll find them useful.

By the way, the guy I mentioned at the beginning did realize that the culprit in him gaining three (3) pounds was his love of brown rice!

MENOPAUSE

Lately, several women readers, who are suddenly finding themselves in the "throes" of menopause, are contacting me. What I continue to find surprising is the degree to which most of them were totally unprepared, and have no idea what is going on!

Let's see if we can offer a little insight to them (and the men in their lives)...

Many things can happen in a woman's body because of the changes in hormone patterns that begin during the menopausal transition. Some women are bothered by only a few symptoms during perimenopause. Others are very uncomfortable, while the rest hardly feel any different. Scientists are still trying to understand how the hormone changes during the menopausal transition may affect a woman's periods and menopausal symptoms.

Menopause is only one of several stages in the reproductive life of a woman. The entire menopause transition is divided into distinct stages known as premature menopause, premenopause, perimenopause, menopause, and postmenopause.

Low levels of estrogen and progesterone bring on menopause and can cause symptoms such as irregular periods, hot flashes, vaginal dryness, memory loss and difficulty concentrating, insomnia and fatigue, frequent urination, and mood swings.

Premature menopause is menopause that occurs before the age of 40, whether it is natural or induced by medical or surgical means. Women who enter menopause early have symptoms similar to those of natural menopause, like hot flashes, emotional problems, vaginal dryness, and decreased sex drive. However, for some women with premature menopause, these symptoms are severe. Also, women who have premature menopause tend to get weaker bones faster than women who enter menopause later in life.

Perimenopause marks the time when your body begins its move into menopause. It includes the years leading up to menopause—anywhere from 2 to 8 years—plus the first year after your final period. There is no way to predict how long preimenopause will last or how long it will take you to go through it. It's a natural part of a woman's life that signals the ending of her reproductive years.

Menopause is a normal change in a woman's life when her period stops. It is often called the "change of life." During menopause, which usually occurs between the ages of 45 and 55, a woman's body slowly makes less of the hormones estrogen and progesterone. A woman has reached menopause when she has not had a period for 12 months in a row, and there are no other causes for this change.

Eighty-five percent of the women in the United States experience hot flashes of some kind as they approach menopause and for the first year or two after their periods stop. Hot flashes are mostly caused by the hormonal changes of menopause, but can also be affected by lifestyle and medications. A diminished level of estrogen has a direct effect on the part of the brain (hypothalamus) responsible for controlling your appetite, sleep cycles, sex hormones, and body temperature. Somehow, the drop in estrogen confuses the hypothalamus—which is sometimes referred to as the body's "thermostat"—and makes it read "too hot."

The brain responds to this report by broadcasting an all-out alert to the heart, blood vessels, and nervous system: "Get rid of the heat!" This message is delivered instantly. Your heart pumps faster, the blood vessels in your skin dilate to circulate more blood to radiate off the heat, and your sweat glands release sweat to cool you off even more.

This heat-releasing mechanism is how the body keeps from over-heating in the summer, but when the process is triggered instead by a drop in estrogen, your brain's confused response can make you very uncomfortable. Some women's skin temperature can rise six degrees during a hot flash.

Together with progesterone, another female hormone made by the ovaries, estrogen regulates the changes that occur with each monthly period and prepares the uterus for pregnancy. Prior to menopause, the ovaries make more than 90% of the estrogen in a woman's body. Other organs (including the adrenal glands, liver, and kidneys) also make small amounts of estrogen. That's why women continue to have low levels of estrogen after menopause. Because fat cells can also make small amounts of estrogen, women who are overweight when they are going through menopause may have fewer problems with hot flashes and osteoporosis (both of which are re-lated to lack of estrogen).

Headaches are one of the most common and disturbing symptoms women can suffer from during menopause. Menopause migraines & headaches can last between 4 to 72 hours. Anxiety and other forms of emotional daily stress, overwork and fatigue can cause menopause migraines & headaches. Because the most probable cause of migraines & headaches during menopause is hormone imbalance, it is generally felt that declining estrogen hormones are responsible for these migraines and headaches. In short, when hormones fluctuate, blood vessels in the brain overreact, causing headaches and migraines.

Therefore, when estrogen hormones start dropping, it is very probable that migraines will become more frequent and more intense. This can happen in menopause or even when a woman has her normal periods (in which hormonal fluctuations also occur). Therefore, the best way to avoid migraines & headaches during menopause is to keep a healthy balanced level of estrogen hormones.

Although there is very little scientific evidence to support the effectiveness of "natural" therapies for menopausal symptoms, it is possible that some "natural" therapies may provide some relief to women during the menopausal transition. Here are two important points to keep in mind if you are considering these therapies:

- Tell your health care providers about any complementary and alternative practices you use. Give them a full picture of what you do to manage your health. This will help ensure coordinated and safe care.
- "Natural" does not automatically mean "safe." As noted earlier, botanical and other dietary supplements can interact with

each other and with prescription and over-the-counter drugs, affecting how the body reacts.

There is a direct relationship between the lack of estrogen during perimenopause and menopause and the development of osteoporosis.

One of the most important demographic aspects of osteoporosis is that it occurs more in cities of first world countries like the US, the UK and Canada, where people eat dairy products and red meat. There are several theories suggesting that the artificially treated milk and other dairy products are not digested the way they should be. Moreover, when a woman adds red meat to our diet, it may cause leaching way of calcium from her bones and teeth. Thus, making our bones porous and fragile.

There is substantial evidence that eating protein rich diet is also not good for our bones. These eating practices are not common in third world countries and in rural areas where people follow traditional way of life and eat traditional leafy vegetables. Hence, the percentage of people suffering from osteoporosis in third world countries is lower than in developed countries. Osteoporosis is lowest in South African countries where people eat more leafy vegetables and less dairy products.

Apart from this, women particularly in developed countries consume more alcohol and their diet is rich in meats, white flour and dairy products which include cheese and butter. Women's in western countries also smoke. Smoking leads to increased bone mass loss. Smoking also impairs the action of estrogen, which naturally protects bone mass. There is plenty of evidence that smoking causes a significant increase in the risk of development of osteoporosis.

Women who are looking for alternative treatments should know that certain lifestyle changes can contribute to healthy aging, including during the menopausal transition. For example, quitting smoking, eating a healthy diet, and exercising regularly have been shown to reduce the risks of heart disease and osteoporosis.

WOMEN AND CALCIUM

Osteo is another term for bones. Porosis is another terms for porous. Consequently combining the two terms results in the medical term or condition known as osteoporosis, or 'porous bones.' This results in a fragile bone condition, which is basically a severe reduction in bone density.

When bone loss occurs, this produces the dreaded bone disease known as osteoporosis, which afflicts both women and men in their later years. Basically, as the bone loses its ability to repair itself, this results in a skeletal system that will begin to thin. Also, it happens when there isn't enough calcium. As calcium from bone is released into the bloodstream, this calcium is needed more by the body in other areas in order to help maintain healthy nerves and a normal heartbeat.

When a person is young, there is much collagen in the bone, and so the bone remains pliable. But as a person ages, less of the collagen is present, and the bones consequently become more brittle.

Bones are in a constant state of change, while one set of bone cells build new bone tissue, another set of cells breaks bone down. During the growth periods of your teens, the bone-building cells dominate, but as you approach your thirties the cells responsible for bone breakdown start to gain ground which means you begin to lose around .5 percent of your bone mass ever year.

Throughout a lifetime, women lose up to 45-50% and men, 20-30% of bone mass (around 300 mg calcium per day). Our ability to absorb calcium decreases with age; growing children can absorb as much as 75% of dietary calcium while adults absorb around 15%, that's why they need to increase calcium intake through diet or supplements.

For years, women have been told to "bone up" on calcium to prevent osteoporosis, but now this so-called miracle mineral is also being touted for its potential to promote weight loss, relieve depression and anxiety associated with premenstrual syndrome, control high blood pressure, and ward off strokes.

As new evidence points to the elevated role of calcium in preventing disease, it makes sense to get enough of this vital nutrient each day, especially as mid-life approaches. Experts say there is literally no body system that doesn't benefit from a healthy dose.

Here's how the evidence it stacks up:

When looking at mid-life weight gain women with the highest calcium intakes don't gain weight and those with the lowest do.

Because calcium plays a key role in metabolic disorders linked to obesity and insulin resistance, a diet low in calcium literally stockpiles fat cells while a higher calcium diet depletes them. A high calcium diet released a hormone which sends signals that are read by the body's fat cells to lose weight.

Calcium supplementation can relieve the physical and emotional toll of PMS by almost 50%. Women on the high calcium diet are less irritable, weepy, and depressed and averted backaches, cramping, and bloating.

In some people, an increase in calcium consumption can help control blood pressure without anti-hypertensive medication. A high-calcium regimen reduces levels of total cholesterol by and slashes "bad" LDL cholesterol by 11 percent. So-called "good" HDL cholesterol levels remain unchanged.

A 1999 Harvard study reported that calcium supplementation protects against stroke in middle-aged women. Women taking at least 400 mg of calcium supplements had a 12% lower risk of ischemic stroke (the type caused by plaque buildup in blood vessel walls). Dietary calcium, especially in dairy foods, reportedly reduced stroke risk, along with potassium.

Osteoporosis strikes more than seven million Americans, mostly Asian and white women, with another 17 million at serious risk of developing fragile bones that easily collapse, a crippling curving of the spine, and hip fractures. Research shows that boosting calcium intake can halt bone loss, especially when combined with vitamin D, which enhances its absorption.

Calcium may protect against growths that become malignant in those prone to colorectal cancer. Dr. Martin Lipkin, a professor of medicine at Cornell University, who first discovered the link between calcium and colorectal cancer, stresses that both calcium-rich foods and calcium supplements will produce the same beneficial effects.

Osteoporosis is due to several causes. Basically if the body is inefficient in its calcium absorption, this will result in bone loss. The lack of certain vitamins and minerals will also contribute to bone loss. Among these are Vitamin D, Vitamin C, and Vitamin K. The right balance of magnesium and phosphorus can also affect the proper formation of bone density. Even chlorinated water can encourage calcium loss in the body.

Phosphorous found in most soft drinks will affect the calcium/phosphorous balance in the body and may have an adverse effect on calcium absorption. This is one reason why it would be wise to limit the consumption of these drinks, especially if signs of osteoporosis are present.

Osteoporosis is preventable, and if already present can be slowed down to some degree by incorporating the proper diet and eating habits. A supplemental regime of vitamins and minerals, and a regular exercise program that involves some form of weight bearing exercise such as walking or weight lifting.

Going outside every day when possible and thereby getting enough sunshine ensures that Vitamin D from the sunlight is taken into the body as this also will help in the absorption of calcium by the body.

If you have osteoporosis, there are many medications on the market that help to prevent further bone loss and can actually help to rebuild bone mass. Your doctor can guide you through the choices available. The main thing to remember is that prevention is the ideal course of action to fight osteoporosis. Weight-bearing exercises, a good diet, and calcium intake of about 1500 mg a day go a long way in helping your bones, regardless of whether you have or have had hyperthyroidism.

ANTIBIOTIC "SEASON"

A s winter approaches we begin to see the return of cold and flu. What better time to visit the issue of **ANTIBIOTICS**.

As many of us prepare to bombard our doctors for a prescription of antibiotics to deal with colds and flu, let's make sure we understand a little more about antibiotics and the way they work in our bodies.

Antibiotics are responsible for saving millions of lives; there's no question about it. Many of us have had illnesses in the course of our lives where without the use of an antibiotic therapy, we would not still be here!

Before the introduction of antibiotics (penicillin was discovered in 1928), infection was the leading cause of death in America. Once they hit the scene, they were deemed so miraculous, doctors and patients alike saw them as a cure for every condition, serious or not.

However, there is a dark side to these "wonder drugs". As a result of being misused, new generations of disease strains resistant to antibiotic attack have emerged. If this trend continues, we will find ourselves back in the days when even the simplest infection could kill.

INFORMATION IS THE BEST MEDICINE

Just today, a colleague approached and said she was not felling well. Sore throat; headache, the works. She was rushing to a quickly scheduled doctor's appointment. Jokingly, I told her that I would "doctor' her up. She looked me in the eye and said, "don't you think I need an antibiotic?"

Immediately, I asked her if she had a bacterial or viral infection. She wondered why I asked such a question. I informed her that if it were a viral infection, an antibiotic would be useless. " Oh, I guess I need to find that out first before I conclude that I need an antibiotic", she said.

Here you have a classic example of the attitude of many of us, which has led to a serious problem in our world.

I mean it's crazy!

Have a sore throat? Take **penicillin**.

Does the baby have an ear infection? Give her **amoxicillin.**

Do you have a nasty cough and/or cold? Take **erythromycin.**

We have grown so accustomed to taking antibiotics that we <u>demand</u> them whether our condition would actually respond to antibiotic therapy or not. All of the "old-fashioned" cures for colds – bed rest, warm drinks, good nutrition, and other tried and true home remedies – are now considered out of style. It doesn't matter that antibiotics are useless (and even harmful) against viruses. As patients we beg for them, and many doctors give in.

To meet this insatiable demand, pharmaceutical companies responded by flooding the market with new and stronger antibiotics.

We thought we had won the war on infection. We had driven those bugs and germs into full retreat. But they were not to be defeated!

168

Antibiotic "Season"

Just as a rebel army that grows more fearsome after it is driven into the hills, the bugs come back. In true military fashion, they test the antibiotics and find their weak points. The bugs developed new and more powerful weapons, now it is us who are truly on the defensive.

How did all this come to be?

When we use antibiotics to treat low-grade infections it is like using a nuclear warhead to squash the schoolyard bully. It is overkill to the **nth degree**, yet it doesn't get rid of the problem. Just like another bully hiding around the corner, there's always another strain of bacteria ready to pounce when we least expect.

Antibiotics are not foolproof- they kill most but not all of the offending bacteria. The strongest of the bacteria survive and reproduce at exponential proportions, and soon, "smart" strains of bacteria immune to the antibiotic are flourishing. **The stronger the antibiotic, the stronger the surviving bacteria.** To make matters worse, countless numbers of Americans have misused antibiotics by not taking the full course, stopping their medication as soon as they feel better. In so doing, they helped create new and more powerful **superbugs**. Americans also use – or rather overuse – antibacterial soaps and skin products, going so far as to antibacterial additives in children's toys!

All we are doing is making sure that the strongest and most resistant of the deadly bacteria survive and thrive.

What's even deeper is that, even if you take them only when needed and never abuse them, you may be taking antibiotics without even knowing it.

Around 30% of the antibiotics sold in the United States are fed

to livestock, and find their way into the meat and dairy products we eat, as well as water and soil we depend on. Just think about it, every time you eat a piece of meat or drink a glass of milk, you could be consuming minute amounts of antibiotic residue. If scientist tried to intentionally create the "ultimate germ", they couldn't do a better job.

I'm not trying to scare you. The risk of being wiped out by a virulent infection is slight, and the chance that you'll die of an antibiotic-resistant strain of bacteria is slim. Nevertheless, there are some serious costs to the overuse of antibiotics that affect us all.

Have you ever noticed how you often relapse into an illness immediately after taking an antibiotic? It's not your imagination. Antibiotics can actually **weaken** your immune system, leaving you more vulnerable to the next "bug" that comes your way.

Taking an antibiotic for common ailments that can heal on their own is particularly bad for children. (For example, the common cold has an average life of 3-5 days; the standard course of antibiotics is 5-7 days) What many parents may not realize is that the immune system learns through experience. Each encounter with a virus or bacteria teaches immune cells valuable lessons that will be used the next time they meet up with the same "bug". So when children are given antibiotics for every sniffle, they may be robbed of their ability to effectively fight infection on their own. Yes, it may take a day or two longer for children to beat an infection without an antibiotic, but in the long run, it may be far better for the child.

Antibiotics weaken our immune system in another important way that affects both children and adults: These powerful drugs don't just kill the bad bacteria that make us sick, they also affect the billions of "friendly" bacteria that keeps us well. Without these friendly bacteria, we can't digest our food properly or keep our other systems running well. The side effects of antibiotics are limited to a little indigestion. Antibiotics wipe out the good bacteria that keep us from getting overwhelmed by harmful **E. coli infections, salmonella, and staph.** Overuse of antibiotics has resulted in an epidemic of yeast infections in women. Many strains of yeast are now drug resistant, too!

The overuse of antibiotics has created a new breed of smarter and more virulent bacteria that are practically indestructible. For example, *Streptococcus pneumoniae* – the most common cause of bacterial ear infections in young children – has grown resistant to standard doses of **amoxicillin**, the first line of treatment. Drug-resistant **staph** infections – once easily cured with penicillin- run rampant throughout the nation's hospitals. What I find even more frightening is the recent discovery of **staph** bacteria that are resistant to **vancomycin**, the most powerful antibiotic on the planet!

All of this is more reason to take care of your immune system. When your immune system functions well, it can usually take care of little problems before they become big ones.

After all, a little tolerance can go a log way in dealing with colds, which tend to run their course in 3-5 days, or the flu that generally is history after 7-10 days. A good diet, plenty of rest, and lots of fluids can, in many cases, make the process more bearable.

THE IMMUNE SYSTEM

Inside your body there is an amazing protection mechanism called the immune system. It is designed to defend you against millions of bacteria, microbes, <u>viruses</u>, toxins and parasites that would love to invade your body. To understand the power of the immune system, all that you have to do is look at what happens to anything once it dies. That sounds gross, but it does show you something very important about your immune system.

When something dies, its immune system (along with everything else) shuts down. In a matter of hours, all sorts of bacteria, microbes, and parasites... invade the body None of these things are able to get in when your immune system is working, but the moment your immune system stops the door is wide open. Once you die it only takes a few weeks for these organisms to completely dismantle your body and carry it away, until all that's left is a skeleton. Obviously your immune system is doing something amazing to keep all of that dismantling from happening when you are alive.

The immune system is complex, intricate and interesting. And there are at least two good reasons for you to know more about it. First, it is just plain fascinating to understand where things like fevers, hives, inflammation, etc., come from when they happen inside your own body. You also hear a lot about the immune system in the news as new parts of it are understood and new drugs come on the market — knowing about the immune system makes these news stories understandable.

Your immune system works around the clock in thousands of different ways, but it does its work largely unnoticed. One thing that causes us to really notice our immune system is when it fails for some reason. We also notice it when it does something that has a side effect we can see or feel. Here are several examples:

- When you get a cut, all sorts of bacteria and viruses enter your body through the break in the skin. When you get a splinter you also have the sliver of wood as a foreign object inside your body. Your immune system responds and eliminates the invaders while the skin heals itself and seals the puncture. In rare cases the immune system misses something and the cut gets infected. It gets inflamed and will often fill with pus. Inflammation and pus are both side effects of the immune system doing its job.
- When a mosquito bites you, you get a red, itchy bump. That too is a visible sign of your immune system at work.
- Each day you inhale thousands of germs (bacteria and viruses) that are floating in the air. Your immune system deals with all of them without a problem. Occasionally a germ gets past the immune system and you catch a cold, get the flu or worse. A cold or flu is a visible sign that your immune system failed to

stop the germ. The fact that you get over the cold or flu is a visible sign that your immune system was able to eliminate the invader after learning about it. If your immune system did nothing, you would never get over a cold or anything else.

- Each day you also eat hundreds of germs, and again most of these die in the saliva or the acid of the stomach. Occasionally, however, one gets through and causes food poisoning. There is normally a very visible effect of this breach of the immune system: vomiting and diarrhea are two of the most common symptoms.

- There are also all kinds of human ailments that are caused by the immune system working in unexpected or incorrect ways that cause problems. For example, some people have allergies. Allergies are really just the immune system overreacting to certain stimuli that other people don't react to at all. Some people have diabetes, which is caused by the immune system inappropriately attacking cells in the pancreas and destroying them. Some people have rheumatoid arthritis, which is caused by the immune system acting inappropriately in the joints. In many different diseases, the cause is actually an immune system error.

- Finally, we sometimes see the immune system because it prevents us from doing things that would be otherwise beneficial. For example, organ transplants are much harder than they should be because the immune system often rejects the transplanted organ. When the foreign tissue is placed inside your body, its cells do not contain the correct identification. Your immune system therefore attacks the tissue. The problem cannot be prevented, but can be diminished by carefully matching the tissue donor with the recipient and by using immunosuppressing drugs to try to prevent an immune system reaction. Of course, by suppressing the immune system these drugs open the patient to what are known as opportunistic infections.

Sometimes the immune system makes a mistake. One type of mistake is called autoimmunity: the immune systems for some reason attacks your own body in the same way it would normally attack a germ. Two common diseases are caused by immune system mistakes. Juvenile-onset diabetes is caused by the immune system attacking and eliminating the cells in the pancreas that produce insulin. Rheumatoid arthritis is caused by the immune system attacking tissues inside the joints.

Allergies are another form of immune system error. For some reason, in people with allergies, the immune system strongly reacts to an allergen that should be ignored. The allergen might be a certain food, or a certain type of pollen, or a certain type of animal fur. This reaction is caused primarily by mast cells in the nasal passages. In reaction to the pollen the mast cells release histamine. Histamine has the effect of causing inflammation, which allows fluid to flow from blood vessels. Histamine also causes itching. To eliminate these symptoms the drug of choice is, of course, an antihistamine.

TO VACCINATE OR NOT?

Vaccination is a controversial subject, and many parents worry about subjecting their children to them. Vaccines have caused a lot of controversy in recent years, often confusing—and scaring—parents about the pros and cons of immunizations. Should you vaccinate your child and protect her from more than a handful of infectious diseases, or are the shots themselves more harmful than helpful?

For some children, starting school will trigger the discussion because of school requirements for vaccinations.

How do you make the decision? What do you really understand? Well, here's a little information to help you in the process.

Now that vaccines have virtually eliminated many once-feared diseases, the possibility of vaccine side effects or adverse reactions loom larger in some people's minds than the diseases that vaccines prevent. Most parents today have never seen a case of diphtheria or measles, and some wonder why their children must receive so many shots. Rumors and misinformation about vaccine safety abound. For example, many parents are concerned that multiple vaccines may weaken or overwhelm an infant's immune system or that certain vaccines may cause autism, multiple sclerosis, or diabetes.

By the mid-1980s, there were seven vaccines: diphtheria, tetanus, pertussis, measles, mumps, rubella and polio. Because six of these vaccines were combined into two shots (DTP and MMR), and one, the polio vaccine, was given by mouth, children still received five shots by the time they were 2 years old and not more than one shot at a single visit. Since the mid-1980s, many vaccines have been added to the schedule. Now, children could receive as many as 24 shots by 2 years of age and five shots in a single visit. The result is that the vaccine schedule has become much more complicated than it once was, and children are receiving far more shots than they ever did.

Adolescents, like adults, were recommended to get tetanus boosters every 10 years; most requiring their first booster dose around age 11. Other than this, however, most adolescents did not require additional vaccines unless they missed one in childhood. By 2005, vaccines specifically recommended for adolescents were only recommended for sub-groups of adolescents based on where they lived or medical conditions that they had. However, a new group of vaccines has become available in the latter part of the decade. Vaccines for meningococcus and human papillomavirus (HPV) as well as expanded recommendations for influenza now provide opportunities for adolescents to be protected as they enter their teenage years.

Infectious disease was the leading cause of death in children 100 years ago, with diphtheria, measles, scarlet fever, and pertussis accounting for most them. Today the leading causes of death in children less than five years of age are accidents, genetic abnormalities, developmental disorders, sudden infant death syndrome, and cancer.

Certainly, the number of vaccinations recommended for children has mushroomed over the past two decades. In 1985, children were vaccinated for seven diseases. Now, that number is 16.

What this means is that a child can receive as many as 30 shots by age 6!

Most parents dutifully take their infants to the doctor or clinic at the prescribed times to be vaccinated. Generally, it doesn't occur to them to question this public health institution. However, growing numbers of doctors, scientists and parents have become suspicious about the long-term implications of what some consider a national experiment posturing as solid science. In many ways, the development of immunization theory has been compromised by the theory's very successes.

The history of vaccines does indeed have some glorious chapters. In 1796, British country doctor Edward Jenner formulated a vaccine that led to the global eradication in our time of the deadly smallpox virus. A century later, French chemist Louis Pasteur formulated a vaccine against rabies and even foresaw serums made from nonliving substances that would one day materialize as synthetic, chemical vaccines.

To understand how vaccines teach your body to fight infection, let's first look at how the immune system fends off and learns from a naturally occurring infection. Then we'll examine how vaccines mimic this process.

Imagine you are a dockworker on the piers of Philadelphia. The year is 1793. As you are unloading crates of tea and spices from an oceangoing ship, a mosquito bites you on the arm. This mosquito carries the virus that causes yellow fever, which the mosquito picked up when it bit a sailor who recently returned from Africa. So now you have thousands of yellow fever viruses swarming into your body. In fact, you have become part of an infamous epidemic that will claim the lives of 10 percent of the people in Philadelphia, and all that stands between you and a fatal case of yellow fever is your immune system.

Your immune system is a complex network of cells and organs that evolved to fight off infectious microbes. Much of the immune system's work is carried out by an army of various specialized cells, each type designed to fight disease in a particular way. The invading viruses first run into the vanguard of this army, which includes big and tough patrolling white blood cells called macrophages (literally, "big eaters"). The macrophages grab onto and gobble up as many of the viruses as they can, engulfing them into their blob-like bodies.

While your immune system works to rid your body of yellow fever, you feel awful. You lie in bed, too dizzy and weak even to sit up. During the next several days, your skin becomes yellow (or jaundiced) and covered with purple spots. You vomit blood. Your doctor looks grim and tired: He knows that as many as 20 percent of people who contract yellow fever die, and the epidemic is spreading fast through the city.

You are one of the lucky ones, though. After about a week, your immune system gains the upper hand. Your T cells and antibodies begin to eliminate the virus faster than it can reproduce. Gradually, the virus disappears from your body, and you feel better. You get out of bed. Eventually, you go back to working the docks. If you are ever bitten by another mosquito carrying the yellow fever virus, you won't get the disease again. You won't even feel slightly sick. You have become immune to yellow fever because of another kind of immune system cell: memory cells. After your body eliminated the disease, some of your yellow-fever-fighting B cells and T cells converted into memory cells. These cells will circulate through your body for the rest of your life, ever watchful for a return of their enemy. Memory B cells can quickly divide into plasma cells and make more yellow fever antibody if needed. Memory T cells can divide and grow into a yellow-fever-fighting army. If that virus shows up in your body again, your immune system will act swiftly to stop the infection.

Vaccines teach your immune system by working in the same way and mimicking a natural infection.

No vaccine is perfectly safe or effective. Each person's immune system works differently, so occasionally a person will not respond to a vaccine. Very rarely, a person may have a serious adverse reaction to a vaccine, such as an allergic reaction that causes hives or difficulty breathing. But serious reactions are reported so infrequently—on the order of 1 in 100,000 vaccinations—that they can be difficult to detect and confirm. More commonly, people will experience temporary side effects, such as fever, soreness, or redness at the injection site. These side effects are, of course, preferable to getting the illness.

The decision to vaccinate your child is a personal one. Whatever you decide, it's important that you have enough information to make a good decision…one you can live with. Hope this helps!

SWINE FLU, EPIDEMICS, VIRUSES AND OTHER THINGS

W̲e seem now to hear talk about the Flu year-round in recent years. Whether the topic is seasonal influenza, bird flu or something called a pandemic, everyone seems to be searching for answers about how to avoid them all. One of your best defenses is to understand them.

The flu, more scientifically known as influenza, is a highly contagious respiratory infection caused by influenza viruses. The influenza virus usually enters the body through mucus membranes in the mouth, nose or eyes. When a person with the flu coughs or sneezes, the virus then becomes airborne and can be inhaled by anyone nearby.

According to the CDC, about 5% to 20% of Americans get the flu each year. More than 200,000 people are hospitalized, and about 36,000 people die.

Information is the Best Medicine

Viruses, like the ones responsible for the Flu, are strange things that straddle the fence between the living and the non-living. On the one hand, if they're floating around in the air or sitting on a doorknob, they're harmless. They're about as alive as a rock. But if they come into contact with a suitable plant, animal or bacterial cell, they spring into action. They infect and take over the cell like pirates hijacking a ship. Viruses exist for one purpose only: to reproduce. To do that, they have to take over the reproductive machinery of the host cells.

Viruses are so small in fact, that the largest virus is equal in size to the smallest bacteria. One cell can be used to create thousands of new, mature viruses. They work fast as well. In fact, the fastest virus only needs 24 minutes to invade a cell and release new virus particles.

Recently, the CDC reported an April outbreak of swine influenza originating in Mexico and appearing in California and Texas. Influenza epidemics may occur at any time, but they are more likely in the winter and early spring. Typically, April and May are not true large epidemic outbreak months. Nevertheless, as of April 24, 2009 there have been a total of over 1,004 cases in Mexico with 20 deaths.

Each year there are new strains, new vaccines and new fears of influenza. Medicine has produced definitive vaccines for polio, measles, mumps, smallpox, chickenpox, hepatitis, and even papilloma viruses. Yet, there is no single effective vaccine for influenza. The CDC recommends that, "In general, anyone who wants to reduce their chances of getting influenza can get vaccinated."

While a number of research studies have demonstrated that flu vaccination works, the effectiveness of the flu vaccine can vary from year to year and among different groups of people. The ability of a flu vaccine to

Swine Flu, Epidemics, Viruses and Other Things

protect a person depends on at least two things: 1) The age and health status of the person getting the vaccine and 2) The similarity or "match" between the virus strains in the vaccine and those in circulation.

There are three main types of flu virus, and each type can mutate, or change, from year to year. Thus, there are literally thousands of possible strains. (Each strain is thoroughly analyzed and given a name, often a title associated with the place where it was initially discovered.) Every year health officials produce a new flu vaccine containing three mutated strains of flu virus. To determine which strains to use, US officials, at the beginning of the year, assess circulating flu viruses around the world. They try to guess which strains will reach the United States by the end of the year. Production begins, and the new vaccine is usually available by October, in time for the beginning of the "Flu season".

Influenza viruses are designated as type A, B, or C. Influenza A and influenza B viruses are responsible for most outbreaks of the flu. Influenza A viruses usually cause more extensive and severe outbreaks. While type B viruses affect only humans, influenza A viruses affect many different species (humans, birds, pigs, horses, even dogs). Influenza C viruses result in mild respiratory illnesses and are not believed to cause flu outbreaks.

The flu vaccine traditionally contains two or three inactive or "dead" viruses (out of a possible 200 flu strains) that were prevalent the year before. But, since these strains are constantly changing, vaccinations are only partly successful in preventing outbreaks of the disease. In other words, medical science is constantly playing catch-up, hoping that last year's strains match those in circulation this year.

So what do you need to know about how can you protect yourself?

You should seek medical attention if have a fever of 102 or if you feel very sick. Swine flu has flu-like symptoms of lethargy or muscle aches or pains. And no, previous flu shots do not provide any protection from this disease. No matter how many times in your life before that you've had the flu, that doesn't provide any protection, either.

That's one of the many reasons everyone is so concerned about this strain.

Take good care of yourself and live the best life possible!

COCKROACHES, ASTHMA, AND CHILDREN

For many people the mere mention of the word *"cockroach"* makes one's hair stand on edge. We associate these small insects with indoor dirt and decay, and we know how hard it can be to rid one's home of an infestation of roaches once they settle in. But roaches are a fact of modern urban and suburban life. For some of us, exposure to roaches is an important cause of our asthma. For all of us, an important lesson can be learned from understanding the emerging information about the relationship between cockroach exposure and asthma.

Cockroaches are some of the nastiest bugs to have invading your home. In the summer, they present a much larger indoor problem than they do in the cooler spring and fall months. Too much heat outside actually drives the cockroaches indoors, causing them to seek out the moist areas of your home.

INFORMATION IS THE BEST MEDICINE

Cockroaches are insects with 6 legs and 2 pairs of wings that are common throughout the United States, but especially in the South and in crowded cities. Cockroaches give off proteins, mainly in their saliva and droppings that trigger strong allergic reactions. In roach-infested apartments, these so-called antigens are densest in the kitchen, but they get tracked into other rooms and become ground into rugs and furniture.

Asthma is a growing concern in this country, particularly in inner-city African-American and Latino populations. Inner city children have the highest prevalence and the highest mortality rates for asthma in the United States. Children exposed to high levels of air pollution during their first year of life run a greater risk of developing asthma, pollen allergies, and impaired respiratory function.

The nasty, lowly cockroach has been found to be the leading cause of severe childhood asthma in the country's poorest city neighborhoods, like those throughout Philadelphia, where asthma is worst.

Asthma is on the rise in cities and suburbs alike, but it is especially bad in the inner cities, with rates often double those found elsewhere. A major study attempted to learn the reason for this burden. It found that cockroaches are the most common trigger of inner-city asthma, and children who live in roach-infested homes have the most severe cases.

When most people think of allergy "triggers," they often focus on plant pollens, dust, animals and stinging insects. In fact, cockroaches also can trigger allergies and asthma. In the 1970s, studies made it clear that patients with cockroach allergies develop acute asthma attacks. The attacks occur after inhaling cockroach allergens and last for hours. Asthma has steadily increased over the past 30 years. It is the most common chronic disease of childhood. Now we know that the frequent hospital admissions of inner-city children with asthma often is directly related to their contact with cockroach allergens—the substances that cause allergies. From 23 percent to 60 percent of urban residents with asthma are sensitive to the cockroach allergen.

To the surprise of many, as far back as 1997, a large study supported by the National Institute of Allergy and Infectious Diseases (NIAID) concluded that the combination of cockroach allergy and exposure to the insects is an important cause of asthma-related illness and hospitalizations among children in U.S. inner-city areas.

Now who can say they knew about this?

Asthma affects about 20 million Americans. Inner-city children (many of them disproportionately African American and Latino) suffer disproportionately from the disease, and exposure to high levels of multiple indoor allergens and tobacco smoke is a contributing factor.

Cockroaches live everywhere, but are found at higher levels in the older, multi-storied, and poorly maintained areas of the inner city. They're a given in year-round tropical climates, but with the prevalence of central heating, roaches can live anywhere in any season. The older the housing the more likely there will be remnants of cockroaches. Studies show that 78 percent to 98 percent of urban homes have cockroaches. Each home has from 900 to 330,000 of the insects.

The study found that children who were both allergic to cockroaches and exposed to high cockroach allergen levels were hospitalized for their asthma 3.3 times more often than children who were allergic but not exposed to high levels of cockroach allergen, or children who were exposed to high levels of cockroach allergen but who were not allergic.

Asthma is the leading cause of school absenteeism due to chronic illness and is the second most important respiratory condition as a cause of home confinement for adults. Each year, asthma causes more than 18 million days of restricted activity, and millions of visits to physicians' offices and emergency rooms. A recent study found that children with asthma lose an extra 10 million school days each year; this problem is compounded by an estimated $1 billion in lost productivity for their working parents.

Children who were both allergic and heavily exposed to cockroach allergen also missed school more often, needed nearly twice as many unscheduled asthma-related medical visits, and suffered through more nights with lost sleep.

Cockroach allergy is more common among poor African Americans. Experts believe that this is not because of racial differences; rather, it is because of the disproportionate number of African Americans living in the inner cities.

Allergic reactions cause asthma symptoms to flare up. This can be annoying for some people and a medical emergency for others. You can help limit flare-ups by reducing contact with your known allergy triggers. Sometimes allergy medicine is prescribed for people with asthma who have allergies. Asthma is a chronic inflammatory disease of the airways that causes shortness of breath, tightness in the chest, coughing and wheezing. During an asthma attack, the airways narrow and become obstructed, making it hard for air to move through – thus making breathing difficult. Asthma can be very scary – and when not controlled, it can be life threatening.

Although allergies and asthma are separate entities, they are related. People who have allergies– particularly allergies that cause symptoms of the nose and eyes – are more likely to have asthma. About 75 percent of children with asthma also have allergies. Many people with asthma find their symptoms get worse when they are exposed to specific allergens. In addition, the conditions tend to run in families, so if you have allergies or asthma, your child is more likely to have one or both of the conditions.

At the end of the day, what makes the statistics about minority children and asthma remarkable is that there is actually no mystery to asthma management. This is not "rocket science". As a society, we need to be committed to improving the living conditions, diets, and the ability to have adequate physical activity. Even though we don't know how to prevent asthma, we really do know how to control the symptoms.

Trivia Fact: There are approximately 5,000 species of cockroaches worldwide!

BACK TO SCHOOL FOR
THE CHILD WITH ADHD

You may hate to admit it, but you are probably looking forward to having your children go back to school. You know that there is a lot to do before school starts, like back-to-school shopping. You also know that for your child who has Attention Deficit Hyperactivity Disorder (ADHD), there may be more to do...

Was your child off of their ADHD medications during the summer break? If so, you may want to restart it at least a week or two before school starts to get back the routine of taking her medicine each day. This is especially important if your child is taking a drug like Strattera, which can take a two or three weeks to even begin working.

Otherwise, the start of school is not a real good time to make any big changes in your child's treatment regimen. Your child will already be faced with new teachers and classes and perhaps a new school and new friends. It may help to give your child a few weeks to adjust to the new year before making any changes to her medication, especially if you are considering stopping her medicine altogether.

It seems that back-to-school time always sneaks up. Before you know it, the summer is over and school is starting again. Helping your child ease from the lazy days of summer to the structured days of fall is important. If your child has ADD / ADHD, transitions can sometimes be difficult. Many children experience mixed feelings about restarting school. School may create feelings of excitement, but it can also create some anxiety, especially if previous school experiences have been frustrating.

No one knows exactly what causes this behavioral disorder. A brain injury may be behind some cases, and environmental and genetic factors could be to blame as well.

In particular, family history seems to play a significant role: 25% of close relatives of those with ADHD may have it too. And for people with a family history, it's possible genetic makeup could increase the odds of one's getting it by as much as 50% to 80%. Take dads, as an example. At least one-third of all fathers who had ADHD in their youth have children with ADHD.

In addition to your child's ADHD medication, other issues to think about as your child goes back to school can include:

Is your child getting enough sleep? Many children with ADHD do not sleep well, which can contribute to hyperactivity, irritability, and a decreased attention span, which many parents may think to blame as a side effect of their ADHD medication or simply on their ADHD.

Does your child need extra help, even as his ADHD medication is helping most of his/her ADHD symptoms? If so, then you might ask your pediatrician to fill out an Other Health Impaired (OHI) form from the Individuals with Disabilities in Education Act (IDEA) to get extra special education services in school or request that the school evaluate him/her under section 504 of the Rehabilitation Act of 1973.

It's important to set the stage for the teacher to see the child as an individual, separate from whatever previous ideas or information they have. It has often been helpful for parent and child to write individual personal letters to teachers as a way to communicate this information. Many families have found letter writing to be a wonderful process that brings the child closer to his or her teachers on a more personal level–a level that facilitates more personal connections between teacher, child and parent. The letter is a chance to present the child as an individual, not just a child with ADHD.

As a parent your letter should include a description of your child, identifying which subtype of ADHD he or she has and specifying the characteristics of that subtype that your child displays. You might also describe what treatment is being used; the people on the treatment team; the treatment itself; including information about behavior plans and medications currently in use and any that have been discontinued. Describe the strategies that you and previous teachers have found to be helpful, such as advance warnings about schedule changes or touch prompts. Also specify techniques that have not worked or even backfired. Include other personal information: your child's likes, dislikes, hobbies, strengths, weaknesses and accomplishments.

Letters such as these enable children to educate their teachers about themselves and their ADHD, rather than waiting for the disorder to manifest itself in a negative context, and they tend to evoke an empathic response from teachers. Try to help your children identify, in his/her own words, what ADHD is, how it affects them, and what helps them to learn best in class.

Back to School for the Child with ADHD

This early and open communication among children, teachers and parents has several benefits:

1. It decreases the time it takes for a new teacher to work effectively with the child.
2. It presents the child as approachable, likable and easier to connect with.
3. It begins the process of open communication.
4. It provides an opportunity to empower children to deal with their ADHD. They can get an early start in advocating for themselves that will serve them well throughout their school years and beyond.

The most important aspect of preparing your child for school is to decrease anxiety and to increase your child's sense of competence. Because most children with ADHD have struggled in school academically, behaviorally, and/or socially, approaching the first days of school can feel overwhelming for children and parents alike. For some children, easing into routines at home for sleep, meals, and after school activities (including homework) can be helpful a week or more before school starts, with the goal of helping the child prepare for these routines and avoiding battles during the early days of school. It's important to emphasize academic strengths and favorite activities, but acknowledge anxieties, as well. Most children do not want to talk about school but will appreciate their parent's acknowledgement of the effort that is involved.

JUNK FOOD AND HEALTH

<hr>

With new mandatory nutritional posting laws taking effect on menus at restaurants and fast food take-out places, it is important to understand why junk food can rob you of good health. This is especially true for our young people.

The latest city ordinance in the country, mandating the posting of nutritional posting in food establishments, is one introduced by Philadelphia Councilwoman Blondell Reynolds-Brown. Even though the new law will go a long way to impact the health dangers of obesity, it serves as an opportunity to address the more far-reaching health risks inherent the prevalence of junk food in our society.

When a teenager's diet consists of junk food and fast foods, it has more fat, sugar and salt than nutrients. This improper diet has both short-term and long-term ill effects on the body.

What's in some of that Junk Food?

- A can of cola contains 10 teaspoons of sugar.
- The metal in the can of soda costs more than the ingredients

(mainly water with additives, refined sugar and caffeine).

- A super-sized order of fries contains 610 calories and 29 grams of fat.
- Artificial ingredients can contain an alarming variety of chemicals. For instance, 'artificial strawberry flavor' can contain about 50 chemicals... and no strawberries at all!
- A king-sized Burger with cheese, large fries and large drink contains 1,800 calories (mostly derived from fat and refined sugar). To 'burn' these calories would take nearly 6 hours of cycling (at 20 miles per hour).

The effects of a constant diet comprised mostly of junk food are not to be ignored. Much of the rise in behavior problems, particularly violence and aggression we are seeing in our young people, may have its' roots in junk food. Increasing rates of anxiety, depression and irritability could be due to a poor diet that lacks the essential chemicals to keep the brain healthy. Changes in diet over the past 50 years appear to be an important factor behind a significant rise in mental ill health.

Several recent reports describe the links between the less severe forms of mental disorder, such as anxiety, and the nation's increasing reliance on ready meals and processed food, which are heavy in pesticides, additives and harmful trans fats. It is a known fact that eating a diet without fresh fruit and vegetables, fish, poultry, or nuts deprives the brain of the essential vitamins and nutrients needed to regulate it.

A report, 'Feeding Minds', produced by the Mental Health Foundation and Sustain, argues that dietary changes could hold the key to combating problems such as depression and ADHD (attention deficit hyperactivity disorder) in children.

INFORMATION IS THE BEST MEDICINE

Over the past 60 years, there has been a significant decline in the consumption of fruit and vegetables, with only 13 per cent of men and 15 per cent of women now eating at least five portions each day. The number of pesticides and additives in food has risen sharply over the same period.

The brain relies on a mixture of complex carbohydrates, essential fatty acids (EFAs)–particularly Omega 3 and Omega 6–vitamins and water to work properly. Highly processed food contains high levels of trans fats–unsaturated oils that have been refined–which can assume the same position in the brain as the EFAs, without delivering the proper nutrients.

Nutritional deficiency could seriously hamper the body's production of amino acids, which are vital to good psychological health. Neurotransmitters, made from amino acids, are chemicals that transmit nerve impulses between the brain cells.

Serotonin, a key neurotransmitter made by the amino acid tryptophan, helps to regulate feelings of contentment and anxiety, as well as playing a role in regulating depression. Many of us do not have sufficient levels of tryptophan because their intake of nuts, seeds and whole grains is too low.

The Mental Health Foundation says scientific studies have clearly linked attention deficit disorder, depression, Alzheimer's disease and schizophrenia to junk food and the absence of essential fats, vitamins and minerals in industrialized diets.

Food can have an immediate and lasting effect on mental health and behavior because of the way it affects the structure and function of the brain. Mental health has been completely neglected by those working on food policy. Rates of depression have been shown to be higher in countries with low intakes of fish, for example. Lack of folic acid, omega-3 fatty acids, selenium and the amino acid tryptophan are thought to play an important role in the illness. Deficiencies of essential fats and antioxidant vitamins are also thought to be a contributory factor in schizophrenia.

Most mental health patients generally have the poorest diets. They are eating lots of convenience foods, snacks, takeaways, chocolate bars, and crisps. It's very common for them to be drinking a liter or two of soda each day. They get lots of sugar but a lot of them are eating only one portion of fruit or vegetable a day, if that.

Researchers at the University of Liverpool examined the toxic effects on nerve cells in the laboratory of using a combination of four common food additives–aspartame, Monosodium glutamate (MSG) and the artificial colorings brilliant blue and Quinoline yellow.

The Liverpool team reported that when mouse nerve cells were exposed to MSG and Brilliant blue or aspartame and quinoline yellow in laboratory conditions, combined

In concentrations that theoretically reflect the compound that enters the bloodstream after a typical children's snack and drink, the additives stopped the nerve cells growing and interfered with proper signaling systems. The mixtures of the additives had a much more potent effect on nerve cells than each additive on its own.

Exposure to food additives during a child's development has been associated with behavioral problems such as attention deficit hyperactivity disorder.

Additives are licensed for use one at a time, but the study's authors believe that examining their effect in combinations gives a more accurate picture of how they are consumed in the modern diet.

Although the use of single food additives is believed to be relatively safe in terms of development of the nervous system, their combined effects are unclear; there are signs that when you mix additives, the effect might be worse.

Brilliant blue is found in sweets, some processed peas, some soft drinks and some confectionery, desserts and ices. Quinoline yellow is found in some sugar products and some pickles. MSG, which should be banned in foods for young children, is found in some pasta with sauce products, a large number of potato chips, processed cheese, and fast food meals. Aspartame is found in diet drinks, some sweets, and desserts and even in some medicines.

BEST CHOICES AND WORST:

Good for the brain:
- Vegetables, especially leafy
- Seeds and nuts
- Fruit
- Whole grains
- Wheat germ
- Organic eggs
- Organic farmed or wild fish, especially fatty fish

Bad for the brain:
- Deep fried junk foods
- Refined processed foods
- Pesticides
- Alcohol

Junk Food and Health

- Sugar
- Tea and coffee
- Some additives

Any food that has poor nutritional value is considered unhealthy and may be called a junk food. A food that is high in fat, sodium, and/or sugar is known as a junk food. Junk food is easy to carry, purchase and consume. Generally, a junk food is given a very attractive appearance by adding food additives and colors to enhance flavor, texture, appearance, and increasing long shelf life.

Remember, junk foods are empty calories. An empty calorie lacks in micronutrients such as vitamins, minerals, or amino acids, and fiber but has high energy (calories).

Since junk food is high in fats and sugars, it is responsible for obesity, dental cavities, Type 2 diabetes and heart diseases

BAD FOODS OUR
CHILDREN EAT

═══════════

I have become increasingly concerned about the health of our young people. As we continue to see higher rates of typical adult health problems like diabetes, high blood pressure and the like in children, it is appalling to know how much of this is the result of the grossly neglect attitude that we, as adults, have in respect to what we have allowed to be commonplace in their diets.

It's no secret that for years, low-income communities of color have suffered as grocery stores and fresh, affordable food disappeared from their neighborhoods. But few of us stop and take note of what this is doing to our children.

Have you ever gone late to work, so you can have breakfast with your child at school to see what they serve? How about remembering the last time you took your child to the supermarket to teach them how to shop for food? When was the last time you looked around a typical corner store, paying attention to what many of our children are eating everyday?

Bad Foods our Children Eat

I recently came across a study that looked at the role of corner stores in our children's lives. Needless to say, it was a sobering insight into just how poorly we have failed our children in providing guidance and protection as they learn the food habits and behaviors that will surely lead to them being unhealthy and unproductive adults.

The study by Temple University's Center for Obesity Research and Education revealed that for a "little more than a dollar" city kids can walk into a typical corner store and fill up with unhealthy calories of low-nutrition junk, and for many, it has become a way of life and gateway to obesity. It found that the average Philadelphia student purchases more than 350 calories on each visit to the corner store–and 29 percent of them shop at corner stores twice a day, five days a week, consuming almost a pounds worth of additional calories each week.

In fact, according to The Food Trust, in communities that lack supermarkets, entire families depend on corner stores for food purchases. The choices at these stores are often limited to packaged food and very little, if any, fresh produce. Corner stores are also frequent destinations for children, many of whom stop daily on the way to and from school for snacks.

In another national survey, fat comprised an average of 35% of total caloric intake in youth aged 2 to 19 years, and almost two-thirds of these youth did not eat recommended amounts of fruits and vegetables.

A 2009 study by the U.S. Department of Agriculture found that 23.5 million people lack access to a supermarket within a mile of their home. A recent multistate study found that low-income census tracts had half as many supermarkets as wealthy tracts. Another multistate study found that eight percent of African Americans live in a tract with a supermarket, compared to 31 percent of whites. On the other hand, for every additional supermarket in a census tract, produce consumption increases 32 percent for African Americans.

Studies have shown that a good breakfast boosts not just student nutrition, but also student achievement and health, and reduces absenteeism and visits to the school nurse. This under-nutrition can affect a child's behavior, school performance and overall cognitive development. Even when a child misses one meal, behavior and academic performances are affected. A hungry child has difficulty learning.

For a school age child, the act of not eating breakfast can lead to fatigue and a diminished attention span. While the body adjusts to decreased blood sugar levels, the brain struggles to perform its function with a minimal supply of nutrients. Children up to the age of ten need to eat every four to six hours to maintain a blood sugar concentration high enough to support the activity of the brain and the nervous system. Most teachers can quickly identify those children who come to school without breakfast. Their heads are on their desks at 10:00 AM-the peak learning hours. This chronic poor nutrition may cause more serious learning deficits.

The effectiveness of school-based nutrition programs and services can be enhanced by outreach efforts in the surrounding community. At the very least, school personnel should be familiar with the health and nutrition resources available through local agencies. Contacts can be made with the health department, community nutrition programs, health centers, local food pantries and fitness programs. Once contacts are established, parents and schools can collaborate with other community agencies to positively influence the health and nutritional status of school-age children.

Bad Foods our Children Eat

Junk food is everywhere and it is being consumed by our students in record quantities. "Junk food" is food which traditionally has no nutritional value. It deprives the body of necessary nutrients and its' over consumption over time leads to obesity, medical problems, and behavioral problems. Some examples are: "Salted snack foods, candy, gum, most sweet desserts, fried fast food and carbonated beverages..."

Junk food consumption is associated with various physical ailments including obesity, Type II diabetes, heart attacks, and decreased life expectancy. Because of junk food, "our children's life expectancy could be lower than our own." Junk food is also a major cause in the 23 percent of American children who are overweight. Fast food and the increasingly available category of junk food are strongly correlated to the "300 percent increase in the rate of U.S. children who are either overweight or obese."

While there are no studies specifically linking meals eaten away from home to academic performance, we do know that poor nutrition during the school day can result in behavioral and learning problems. Chronically undernourished children score poorly on standardized tests, are more irritable and exhibit lower energy levels.

Junk food surrounds our children in a new "toxic food environment" which is made worse by a bombardment of advertisements through media directed at children. Junk foods are altering the structure and function of the human brain while increasing and decreasing insulin levels so quickly that junk food leaves students groggy in class. A child's brain continues to develop through until adulthood; many of the foods that students eat affect the growth of critical areas of their brain. When growth is disrupted, in can cause negative behavior reactions in the classroom. Often times, doctors do not seek the root of the problem (food) but instead they mask the behavioral symptoms with drugs such as Ritalin or Prozac which have their own series of side effects, all while the brain development continues to be damaged.

There are many health benefits associated with good nutrition and physical activity. Eating smart and moving more help children and youth maintain a healthy weight, feel better and have more energy. These positive health benefits have the potential to translate into academic benefits at school. Good nutrition and physical activity nourish the brain and body, resulting in students who are present, on time, attentive

In class, on-task and possibly earning better grades. As students work hard to achieve high academic standards, it is more important than ever that we provide opportunities for them to be active and eat healthy throughout the day.

Families, schools, government and communities must share the responsibility of promoting and supporting children and youth to eat smart and move more. We must save the children...

SAFE SCHOOLS AS A
PUBLIC HEALTH EPIDEMIC

Epidemic: Spreading rapidly and extensively by infection and affecting many individuals in an area or a population at the same time.

Infection : the act or result of affecting injuriously.

While bullies, gangs, weapons, and substance abuse all contribute to the fear experienced by many of today's students, violence in America's neighborhoods and communities cannot be overlooked.

More than ever before, today's schools are serving children from dysfunctional homes, children living in poverty, children of teenage parents, and special education students. Unfortunately, resources to adequately serve the total range of needs presented by these students are becoming increasingly limited. Adequate parental supervision and control of these students has weakened, and many students have diminished respect for all forms of authority, including the authority of school personnel.

As a result, schools are confronted with problems of students possessing weapons, students involved with gang recruitment and rivalry, and students engaged in drug trafficking, both as sellers and buyers. Such problems lead to violent acts in and around schools. In order to create a safe environment that is conducive to learning, schools must implement safety plans and comprehensive prevention programs that address the root causes of violence.

Almost without exception, every major city in America is seeing record numbers of young people; mostly African American males die as a result of gun violence.

Although high-profile school student shootings has increased public concern for student safety, you may be surprised to know that school-associated violent deaths account for less than 1% of homicides among school-aged children and youth.

So you see, this is not a "school problem".

At what point do we start to see this as a public health epidemic? A public health approach treats violence like we treat a disease, like we treat an epidemic.

We can start with the mental health component.

Mental and behavioral health is an essential component of young peoples' overall health and wellbeing. It affects how young people think, feel, and act; their ability to learn and engage in relationships; their self-esteem and ability to evaluate situations, options and make choices. A person's mental health influences their ability to handle stress, relate to other people, and make decisions.

Four million children and adolescents in this country suffer from a serious mental disorder that causes significant functional impairments at home, at school, and with peers. It is estimated that one in 10 children and adolescents suffer from mental illness severe enough to cause some level of impairment. However, in any given year, it is estimated that fewer than one in five of such children receives needed treatment.

Who's calling for increases in mental health services available to these young people?

An alarming 65% of boys and 75% of girls in juvenile detention have at least one mental disorder. We are incarcerating youth with mental disorders, some as young as 8 years old, rather than identifying their disorders early and intervening with appropriate treatment.

Early and effective mental health treatment can prevent a significant proportion of delinquent and violent youth from future violence and crime.

The contribution of social factors to the health problems of young African American men deserves further attention than thus far received.

Young African American men die at a rate that is at least 1.5 times the rate of young white men, and almost three times the rate of young Asian men. While the death rate drops for men ages 25 to 29 for most groups, it continues to rise among African Americans.

Are we silly enough to believe that this is because Young African American men are at the bottom of the evolutionary chain? Have you heard of health disparities?

With any other cause of death where African Americans suffer disproportionately (heart disease, cancer, diabetes), it is universally accepted that education, access, social/economic factors are centrally responsible factors. Why are we ignoring not applying the same logic with the public health epidemic of youth violence?

Information is the Best Medicine

Throughout history, "Epidemics" are commonly thought to involve outbreaks of acute infectious disease, such as measles, polio, or streptococcal sore throat. If this were a Flu epidemic, all sorts of vaccines and preventive measure would be put in place and implemented. Unfortunately, just like the Cholera in Haiti, it gets the headlines for a few days, then a return to business as usual.

We are so consumed and focused on "blaming' public school superintendents and police commissioners across America for not doing enough, we can't see the forest for the trees! We have conveniently put this issue in a neat little box called "youth violence".

Education is one of the strongest predictors of health: the more schooling people have, the better their health is likely to be. Although education is highly correlated with income and occupation, evidence suggests that education exerts the strongest influence on health. More formal education is consistently associated with lower death rates, while less education predicts earlier death. The less schooling people have, the higher their levels of risky health behaviors, such as smoking, being overweight, or having a low level of physical activity. High school completion is a useful measure of educational attainment because its influence on health is well studied, and it is widely recognized as the minimum entry requirement for higher education and well-paid employment. A public health approach focuses on risk factors and protective factors. It does not focus on a reactive response of criminal justice, which makes the threat of punishment a primary deterrent.

Seldom have health and education professionals been in a better position to work together to achieve common goals. Rarely has a single problem contributed to so many adverse social, economic, and health conditions. Our nation's young people deserve no less than a concerted effort to give young people a gateway to lifetime health and success.

Interventions to reduce school dropout rates seek to change individuals, families, schools, school systems, or public policies related to poverty, welfare, or employment.

The problem of youth violence is complex and our response needs to draw on the best that all sectors and disciplines have to offer.

Youth violence and school safety is a **public health problem**. Let's not be in denial.

WATERMELON 101

E ven though Watermelon is the leading U.S. melon crop in terms of acreage, production, and per capita consumption. Most Americans would probably be surprised to learn that African Americans are *underrepresented* as watermelon eaters. Blacks represent about 13 percent of the United States population yet only account for 11 percent of the watermelon consumption. It is possible that many African Americans are reluctant to eat watermelons because they do not want to "validate" the stereotype of the shuffling, dull-witted, clumsy, watermelon-eating Negro.

Native to Africa, it was a valuable and portable source of water for desert situations and when natural water supplies were contaminated. Watermelons were cultivated in Egypt and India as far back as 2500 B.C. as evidenced in ancient hieroglyphics.

Watermelons were brought to China around the 10th century and then to the Western Hemisphere shortly after the discovery of the New World. In Russia, where much of the commercial supply of watermelons is grown, there is a popular wine made from this fruit. In addition to Russia, the leading commercial growers of watermelon include China, Turkey, Iran and the United States.

Today, there are several hundred different cultivars, mostly due to the different needs of regional markets: genetic manipulation has allowed for the cultivation of giant watermelons (the largest weighed in at approximately 262 pounds), as well as seedless varieties (derived from cross-pollinating a tetraploid plant with a diploid variety, resulting in a triploid plant with much fewer seeds than normal watermelons). In fact, there are more than 1200 varieties of watermelon ranging in size from less than a pound, to more than two hundred pounds, with flesh that is red, orange, yellow or white.

Watermelons are grown in 44 of the continental United States. If you purchase watermelons in a western state, chances are they were grown in California or Arizona. If you purchase them in a mid-western or eastern state, they are more likely to have been grown in Florida, Georgia, or Texas. If you really crave watermelon for New Year's Day, you can probably get one, since they are imported from Mexico. Domestic melons, however, come into season in May and are around until the end of October. The season's peak is from May through August.

Watermelon is not only a refreshing fruit to beat the heat on a hot summer day but it has a few health advantages. Watermelon is also very effective in reducing your body temperature and blood pressure. Many people in the tropical regions eat the fruit daily in the afternoon during summers to protect themselves from heat stroke. This fruit may also help in reducing inflammation that contributes to conditions like asthma, atherosclerosis, diabetes, colon cancer, and arthritis. Watermelon is full of water, carbohydrates and fiber along with essential vitamins and minerals that provides nutrition to the body for better metabolism.

Watermelon has the highest concentration of lycopene, which is an important antioxidant helpful in fighting heart diseases and cancer. It also contains high amount of potassium, which is essential for muscle nerve function and helps lower blood pressure. The fruit contains vitamin A which helps maintain eye health and is a good antioxidant, B6 provides brain function and vitamin C which helps build immunity and prevent cell damage. They also contain important amino acids citrulline and arginine, which can help maintain arteries, blood flow and overall heart health. The amino acids also improve body's sensitivity towards insulin.

The nutrition of the watermelon doesn't end with the flesh of the fruit. Even though many of spit them out, the seeds aren't necessarily annoying: in some nations of Asia, especially China, roasted seeds are very common and eaten as a snack! Other regions of Africa press them to produce watermelon seed oil, which is common in soups such as egusi. In fact, even the rind is sometimes pickled, or even stir-fried, which means the whole watermelon fruit is edible.

Watermelon seeds are also available in the markets in dried form and have high nutrition in it. The seeds are rich in magnesium and contains high amount of protein and fat. Watermelon seeds are excellent sources of protein (both essential and non-essential amino acids) and oil. Watermelon seed is about 35% protein, 50% oil, and 5% dietary fiber. Watermelon seed is also rich in micro- and macronutrients such as magnesium, calcium, potassium, iron, phosphorous, zinc etc. Scientists know that when watermelon is consumed, a chemical called citrulline is converted to the amino acid known as arginine through certain enzymes. Arginine is an amino acid that works wonders on the heart and circulation system and maintains a good immune system.

The benefits of watermelon don't end there. Arginine also helps the urea cycle by removing ammonia and other toxic compounds from our bodies. Citrulline, the precursor to arginine, is found in higher concentrations in the rind of watermelons than the flesh.

The citrulline-arginine relationship helps heart health, the immune system and may prove to be very helpful for those who suffer from obesity and type 2 diabetes. Arginine boosts nitric oxide, which relaxes blood vessels, the same basic effect that Viagra has, to treat erectile dysfunction and maybe even prevent it.

While there are many psychological and physiological problems that can cause impotence, extra nitric oxide could help those who need increased blood flow, which would also help treat angina, high blood pressure and other cardiovascular problems.

Watermelon may not be as organ specific as Viagra, but it's a great way to relax blood vessels without any drug side effects.

As an added bonus, studies have also shown that deep red varieties of watermelon have displaced the tomato as the lycopene king. Almost 92 percent of watermelon is water, but the remaining 8 percent is loaded with lycopene, an anti-oxidant that protects the human heart, prostate, and skin health.

Ever wonder how they grow seedless watermelons?

A seedless watermelon is a "hybrid", which is created by crossing male pollen for a watermelon, containing 22 chromosomes per cell, with a female watermelon flower with 44 chromosomes per cell. When this seeded fruit matures, the small, white seed coats inside contain 33 chromosomes, rendering it sterile and incapable of producing seeds. This is similar to the mule, produced by crossing a horse with a donkey. This process does not involve genetic modification. Genetically modified foods (or GM foods) are foods derived from genetically modified organisms.

So there you have it. Seedless watermelons are just regular watermelons, albeit a relatively younger relative of the traditional seeded watermelon. Despite being the new kid on the block, the seedless watermelon actually outsells its seeded peers by a significant margin. According to the National Watermelon Promotion Board, only 16 percent of watermelon sold in grocery stores has seeds. Ten Years ago, 46 percent of those sold had seeds.

There's an art to choosing the best watermelon that makes all the difference in the world. The National Watermelon Promotion Board offers these three easy tips for choosing a great watermelon:

- Choose a firm, symmetrical fruit that is free of bruises, cuts and dents.
- Before you buy, pick up your melon. The heavier it feels, the better — a good watermelon is 92% water, which makes up most of its weight.
- On the underside of the watermelon there should be a creamy yellow spot from where it sat on the ground and ripened in the sun.

One final bit of advice for the watermelons you will buy this summer. They store much better uncut if you leave them at room temperature. Lycopene levels can be maintained even as it sits on your kitchen floor. But once you cut it, refrigerate. And enjoy!

SUMMER HEALTH TIPS

Here is some great information to help you do your best to get through the summer with nothing more than great memories and lots of fun.

HEAT STRESS

Heat stress can range from mild to life threatening–can affect men and women, regardless of their age. However young children and the elderly are most vulnerable. Babies and infants can't regulate their body temperature well; the elderly may be taking a medicine that adds to heat stress. Athletes are vulnerable because they use a lot of energy and generate a great deal of heat, so they need to stay hydrated. In its milder form, heat stress symptoms include thirst, fatigue and feeling hot. But if the early warning signs are ignored, true heat illness can develop. Heat illnesses start with cramps, progress to heat exhaustion and can become heat stroke.

HEAT CRAMPS

Heat cramps includes cramping in the legs or abdomen, usually accompanied by dizziness, thirst and rapid heartbeat. At least a quart of water or other unsugared drink is recommended. <u>Drinking liquids is the most important step to keeping healthy.</u> Water is best, but lemonade and iced tea are good substitutes.

Heat Exhaustion

Dizziness, nausea, headaches and rapid heartbeat are symptoms of heat exhaustion. At this point, emergency medical attention is necessary.

Heat Stroke

Heat stroke is serious and requires medical attention immediately. It is the result of the body's inability to manage the heat load. The skin is now hot but dry, and the person may be unconscious. This is a medical emergency. Call 911! Good prevention methods are crucial to staying healthy in the heat. Here are some tips:

- if working outside, try to work in the early morning or after 6 p.m. when it is cooler
- if working in a non-air conditioned area, drink a quart of water every hour
- if your diet allows, use extra salt on foods
- consider air conditioned places such as a mall or library
- do not leave children or pets in the car

In the summertime, many people are rushed to the Emergency Room with heat-related illnesses such as heat exhaustion and heat stroke. Here are some simple tips to help you stay cool.

- Do not overexercise in hot weather.
- Wear a hat to protect yourself from the sun.
- Keep a water bottle handy to sip so that you do not have to worry about dehydration.
- Pace yourself if you are going to be working outside under the sun for a long time. Take regular breaks so your body has a chance to cool down.
- Remember, overcast days are just as hot and dangerous as sunny days

Keep in mind that just the way you go about daily activities can make all the difference.

- **Strokes** can happen any season, but is easier to miss in hot weather, until it's too late! Know the stroke warning signs – weakness, numbness or paralysis to the face, arm or leg (especially on one side of the body), sudden blurred or decreased vision, difficulty speaking or understanding speech, dizziness, balance or coordination problems and sudden or severe headache. Get immediate attention.
- Drink, drink, and drink! **Kidney stones** are more common during the summer months because warmer weather causes dehydration and increases concentration of substances in the urine. These substances crystallize to form stones. Increasing fluid intake (3 to 4 quarts of fluid per day) may help keep kidney stones from forming.
- Watch out for rising temperatures! Problems related to the

summer heat are common for older persons. This is especially true for senior citizens with heart disease and other chronic illnesses, and for people who take certain medicines like diuretics (water pills), some types of antidepressants and tranquilizers. The symptoms of heatstroke are not specific but include dizziness, weakness, nausea, headache and a sensation of warmth. Just as people enjoy the warm temperatures of spring and summer, so do bacteria. Be careful not to leave foods out on the counter in warm weather for any length of time. Foods can be breeding grounds for bacteria. These bacteria produce toxins that may be harmful to the digestive system and cause food poisoning. During the warm weather months, eat only well-stored and refrigerated foods and foods that are thoroughly cooked.

- Avoid the midday sun if you have **heart disease** and your doctor has prescribed an exercise program for you. Do your exercises early in the morning or in the early evening when it is not as hot.
- Sunglasses with UV protection can help enhance the eyes' ability to filter out the sun's damaging rays. Choose sunglasses that block 99 to 100 percent of UV radiation (UV-A and UV-B). Be careful of sunglasses that don't specify exactly what amount of UV rays they block.

A final note on children in the hot weather: In the heat, your baby will most likely sweat more and feel like eating less. To make up for fluids lost due to perspiration, be sure that your child increases his or her fluid intake. Since many infants drink less when they are uncomfortable in the heat, it's best to offer the breast or bottle at frequent intervals. Older children should be given water or diluted fruit juices between their usual bottle feedings. Whenever possible, allow time for your child to cool off after coming inside from a hot day before offering food, since the heat can stifle their appetite. If your baby is eating solids, it's a good idea to try feeding your child smaller meals at more frequent intervals. Don't forget to pack water for yourself.

KEEPING YOUR COOL IN
HOT WEATHER

===

After a long cold winter, most of us are anxious to enjoy the warm days of summer. As soon as the sun comes out we are outside working in the garden, enjoying a game of golf, or just taking a nice long walk. Besides planning ahead for the wonderful warm weather activities, people also need to plan ahead to prevent serious problems caused by the heat.

When the weather's hot, your body works overtime trying to keep cool. Excess heat escapes through sweating, exhalation of warmed air, and increased blood flow to the skin. But hot weather can overwhelm those mechanisms, leading to a wide array of uncomfortable symptoms. If nothing is done to remedy these symptoms, serious harm even life-threatening problems can occur.

The human body consists of nearly 70% water; brain tissue is said to consist of about 85 per cent water. This is why drinking 6–8 glasses of water a day helps our body function efficiently. It is estimated that if we lost just one-tenth of the water within our body, we would not be able to stand, let alone walk.

The body loses fluids in a variety of ways:

- when urinating;
- when you vomit or have diarrhea;
- when sweating; and
- from the lungs when you breathe.

Normally, the body cools itself by sweating. If temperatures and humidity are extremely high, however, sweating is not effective in maintaining the body's normal temperature. When this happens, blood chemistry can change and internal organs—including the brain and kidneys—can be damaged.

The circulation in your body helps to dissipate heat, but when the air temperature is higher than 90°F, cooling by sweat is the only way to prevent the body from overheating. Cooling though evaporation, or sweating, is only possible when your body has been provided with enough fluids. Failing to properly hydrate can result in dizziness, fainting, digestive problems and even death.

Dehydration can quickly lead to fatal collapse of the circulatory system because the heart and temperature control systems cannot dissipate the core heat of your body. Your body is a little furnace- pumping blood; breathing and digestive activities all generate heat deep in the core of your body. If you are working in the heat, the activity of the muscles generates even more energy. If you haven't consumed enough fluids to sweat and cool itself, your body core temperature will rise and begin to destroy tissues and organs. Collapse can come on quickly, although the body gives fair warning of the problem, many people fail to react to the warning signs.

As your temperature starts to rise, your hot blood burns your muscles and your muscles hurt and burn. If you continue to exert yourself, your circulation is compromised when you become extremely short of breath and no matter how hard you breathe, you can't catch your breath. If you ignore this sign, your temperature rises above 106 and your brain is damaged, you get a headache, see spots in front of your eyes, hear ringing in your ears, feel dizzy and pass out.

Lack of fluids set you up for heat stroke, so you need to drink fluids all the time when you are in extremely hot weather. You cannot depend on thirst to tell you when you are dehydrated because you won't feel thirsty until you have lost between two and four pounds of fluid and by then, it is too late to catch up on your fluid deficit.

We all hear the phrase; "You should drink plenty of fluids in hot weather. "Plenty of fluids" mean at least 1-1/2 to 2 quarts of fluids daily. This can be water, fruit juice, or fruit-flavored or carbonated drinks. Since aging can cause a decreased thirst sensation, elderly persons should drink water, fruit juices or other fruit drinks at regular intervals during the day, even if they do not feel thirsty. Avoid alcoholic beverages and those containing caffeine. Salt tablets are not substitutes for fluids.

During hot weather, you will need to drink more liquid than your thirst indicates. Even if you remain indoors and limit your activity, your body still needs to replace lost fluids, salt and minerals. Make an extra effort to drink a minimum of six to eight 8 oz. glasses of cool fluids daily. During heavy exercise in a hot environment, drink two to four glasses of cool fluids each hour. Parents should be sure young children get sufficient fluids. If you are on a special fluid-restricted diet or if you take diuretics, ask your physician about fluid intake during hot weather.

Not drinking enough fluids, doing too much on a hot day, spending too much time in the sun or staying too long in an overheated place can cause heat-related illnesses. Know the symptoms of heat disorders and overexposure to the sun, and be ready to give first aid treatment

Heat disorders include sunburn, heat cramps, heat exhaustion and heat stroke. Children are most susceptible to dehydration; the elderly are most likely to suffer from heat stroke.

Sunburn: Symptoms: Skin redness and pain, possible swelling, blisters, fever, headaches. First Aid: Take a shower, using soap, to remove oils that may block pores preventing the body from cooling naturally. If blisters occur, apply dry, sterile dressings and get medical attention.

Heat Cramps: Symptoms: Painful spasms usually in leg and abdominal muscles. Heavy sweating. First Aid: Firm pressure on cramping muscles or gentle massage to relieve spasm. Give sips of water. If nausea occurs, discontinue.

Heat Exhaustion: Symptoms: Heavy sweating, weakness, weak pulse, normal temperature possible, fainting, vomiting, skin cold, pale and clammy. First Aid: Get victim to lie down in a cool place. Loosen clothing. Apply cool, wet cloths. Fan or move victim to air-conditioned place. Give sips of water. If nausea occurs, discontinue. If vomiting occurs, seek immediate medical attention.

Heat Stroke (Sun Stroke): Symptoms: High body temperature (106 degrees Fahrenheit or higher). Hot, dry skin. Rapid, strong pulse. Possible unconsciousness. Victim will likely not sweat. First Aid: Heat stroke is a severe medical emergency. Call emergency medical services or get the victim to a hospital immediately. Delay can be fatal. Move victim to a cooler environment. Try a cool bath or sponging to reduce body temperature. Use extreme caution. Remove clothing. Use fans and/or air conditioners. DO NOT GIVE FLUIDS.

Keep in mind that many people with health problems should be extra cautious about the heat.

People with diabetes often lack the knowledge to effectively manage their diabetes in hot weather.

People with diabetes have limited ability to sweat and are therefore are at an increased risk for heat-related issues, including dehydration, according to the researchers. In a survey of 152 people in Phoenix, nearly 20% said they would not take precautions until temperatures surpassed 100 degrees. However, heat illness can happen at between 80-90 degrees. Only about half of the patients knew what the definition of the heat index (which measures temperature and humidity).

The researchers said that it is important to take precaution because insulin and oral medications may lose their effectiveness at higher temperatures.

Hot weather also increases dangers for people who must take medicine for high blood pressure, poor blood flow, nervousness or depression.

Summer can be fun, and even exciting. Make sure you don't add to the excitement by becoming a statistic.

Be smart, and anticipate what you will need to avoid problems with the heat. The long hot summer is a welcome change from snow and sleet, so enjoy it!

Drink your water!

FASTING

============

Fasting is a natural process that occurs when you do not consume any food for 3 to 5 hours and during sleep.

Over the past few weeks, I have come across lots and lots of folks who are doing a "fast" of one kind or another: Spring cleaning"; Lent Season; The Master Cleanse; the Lemonade Diet; or the up and coming popular favorite, The Daniel Fast".

There are a lot of reasons why people fast. Fasting historically had a religious meaning associated to it. Then it became associated with social protest by people like Ghandi; Martin Luther King; and my main man, Dick Gregory.

Most recently, lots was written about Beyoncé's weight loss (losing 20 pounds in 10 days) on the Master Cleanse for her movie role in "Dreamgirls" where her character first appears on screen as 16 years old, then later as 36.

While it was true that Beyoncé was gorgeous in the movie, 14 pounds lighter and looking 10 years younger for shooting the younger part, there is a lot of information that most people who fast don't have, so I'd like make an attempt to address the topic.

Starting with Beyoncé, the problem is not what was in the diet but what's not. The diet consists of a mixture of purified water spiked with lemon juice, Grade B maple syrup and cayenne pepper. It was popularized in 1976, as a way to cleanse, detox and lose weight. There are no fats, proteins, vitamins or minerals and the only carbohydrate is in the form of sugar. Clinical scientists say that a person on this diet for an extended period of time would start to feel very lethargic and would be unable to concentrate... They will probably end up in hospital, especially people who try it for more than 10 days.

Even though you may have decided to fast, you should be clear that fasting is not accepted by the vast majority of medical doctors and other healthcare providers, including nutritional and dietary experts. These medical doctors and other healthcare providers believe that extended fasting has too many risks, which outweigh any possible benefits. It is only a very tiny minority of healthcare providers who accept water fasting as a valid process.

If you are fasting to lose weight there are some points that you should keep in mind before you start a fast. There are many types of fasting and you will have to find one that suits your requirement. Discuss the benefits of the different types of fasts with your doctor before you decide.

Let's start with water fasts. Now if you are suffering from conditions like hypoglycemia, hyperglycemia, chronic heart problem or schizophrenia then this fast is not advised. When the body is going through water fasting, the heart rests so it is important that you take deep breaths when you stand up to get the heart pumping or you may feel dizzy or feel a black out coming on.

Fasting

A lot of people can handle a juice fast for about 30 days and safely too. But again those who have problems like diabetes, hypothyroidism, hypoglycemia, etc., should not attempt this without first consulting their doctor. Along with the juice fast, people who have these conditions should supplement the fast with bananas and avocado slices every 2-3 hours. Adding some vegetables to the juices will give it high protein power and a source of fiber will give it the required bulk. This will ensure that your blood sugar is regulated. But if your kidneys are not functioning properly then a juice fast is not advised.

Many intestinal experts say we don't need an extreme diet to cleanse our insides.

Your body does a perfectly good job of getting rid of toxins on its own, there's no evidence that these types of diets are necessary or helpful.

While there are medical conditions that interfere with organ function and prevent the body from clearing toxins, healthy people already have a built-in detoxification system — the liver, kidneys, lungs and skin.

And by attempting to flush out the "bad stuff" from our intestines, you're also "flushing out the good bacteria that keep the intestines healthy."

Here's a look at some of the dangers of fasting for weight loss:

1. FASTING FOR WEIGHT LOSS INCREASES STRESS

When you are fasting, your body will go into a self-preservation mode to counter starvation. It will begin to slow down your metabolism and increase the production of cortisol. Cortisol is a stress hormone that is produced by the adrenal glands. When you are suffering from illness or stress, there will be a larger than usual amount of cortisol in your body. A high amount of cortisol can make you feel physically, mentally or emotionally stressed.

2. FASTING DAMAGES YOUR MUSCLES

When you are not taking enough food, the cortisol in your body will try to release certain amino acids from your muscles and convert them to sugar. The sugar will then be fed to the brain, kidneys and red blood cells. The brain can use fats or sugar as fuel, but it usually prefers sugar, and red blood cells need sugar to survive. By releasing amino acids, cortisol is actually breaking down your muscle tissues. Losing muscles can slow down weight loss, because you need muscles to burn excess fat in your body.

3. FASTING LEADS TO INCREASED HUNGER

If you do not consume food for a prolonged period of time, your body will produce fewer thyroid hormones. The loss of thyroid hormones and muscle tissue breakdown will slow down your body's overall metabolism significantly. This consequence becomes evident when you stop fasting and resume normal eating habits. When you begin to fast, your appetite hormones will be suppressed, but they will go into full gear when normal eating resumes, resulting in increased hunger. With slower metabolism and increased appetite, you will begin to gain weight fast.

4. FASTING CAUSES HEALTH PROBLEMS

Prolonged fasting can deplete the supply of essential nutrients in your body, such as carbohydrates, proteins, vitamins, fatty acids, minerals and electrolytes. This can lead to the development of various health problems, including fatigue, headache, dehydration, dizziness, constipation, hypoglycemia, anemia, muscle weakness, gallstones and mental confusion. If you are suffering from some kind of health problem, it is advisable that you do not fast, because you will become more susceptible to the detrimental effects of fasting.

Most people can fast safely, but if you decide to try it it's important to do so under your doctor's supervision. However, there are some people who should not fast including:

- Infants and young children
- People with serious disease conditions
- Pregnant women
- People with Type I diabetics
- People with insufficient kidney function
- People who experience fear about fasting

Although people can quickly drop pounds on these diets, the majority of people regain all the weight they lose on *any* diet, especially the highly restrictive varieties, according to recent research published in American Psychologist, the journal of the American Psychological Association. While people can lose 5 to 10 percent of their weight in the first few months of a diet, up to two-thirds of people regain even more weight than they lost within four or five years, the researchers found.

Cutting back on high-fat foods, eating in moderation and consuming more vegetables and fruits may not seem as glamorous as starving yourself like a celebrity for days, but it's healthier for you in the long run and certainly sexier than rushing to the bathroom all day.

There are many risks to water-only fasting and we want you to be aware of them prior to your decision to undertake a water-only fast. Because you will not be eating any food, you will most certainly experience weakness throughout the water fast, and lose weight. It can take some time after fasting to regain strength. A very common occurrence is dizziness and fainting, especially on rising from a laying or seating position. Other common and unpleasant symptoms are heart arrhythmia, palpitations, dehydration, nausea, vomiting, skin rashes, sore throat, mucus discharge, low back pain, increased menstrual flow, irregular or menstrual cycles, hair loss, gastric irritation, passing of kidney or gall stones and emotional disturbances. There is also the possibility of alterations to your body's basic mechanisms and electrolytes, which could cause heart problems such as a heart attack or vascular problems such as a stroke.

Let me say it again: If you decide you want to fast, it's important to talk with your health care professional so they can monitor you heath before and during the fast.

HELP TO QUIT SMOKING

You already know smoking causes lung cancer, emphysema, and heart disease, but you're still lighting up. Over the years of working with people and their health issues, rarely have I encountered a more difficult issue than smoking. Most smokers really want to quit, but it seems the urge and addictive nature of the habit always wins. If only it wasn't for nicotine! Nicotine has been said to be even more addictive than alcohol, heroin and cocaine, and it can take as few as four cigarettes to develop a lifelong addiction.

Nicotine is the primary drug found in cigarettes that is potentially very addictive. It causes the same physiological changes in brain chemistry that cause an individual to want to use a drug more and more. Nicotine also creates the symptoms of tolerance and withdrawal common in alcohol and other addictive drugs. The cycle of "euphoric recall" (remembering the pleasant feeling the drug induces) and the physical and psychological discomfort that is caused when the drug is stopped make breaking any addiction very difficult. Understanding this makes me never pass judgment on smokers.

231

The body responds immediately to the chemical nicotine in the smoke when an individual is smoking a cigarette. There is an immediate increase in blood pressure, increase in heart rate and in the flow of blood from the heart. The arteries begin to narrow. There is carbon monoxide present in smoke which reduces the amount of oxygen in the blood. This creates an imbalance between the demand for oxygen by the cells and the amount of oxygen the blood can supply the cells.

Nicotine also produces physical and mood-altering effects in the brain that are both pleasing and calming for many individuals. This calming, pleasant effect reinforces the continued use of nicotine and then the ensuing dependence. The dependence on nicotine is based on both psychological and physical factors. For instance, the smoker develops certain typical behaviors associated with smoking. Usually, a cigarette is smoked after eating, while drinking a cup of coffee or alcohol, in stressful situations or when another smoker is smoking.

As far back as 1988, The Surgeon General's Report, "Nicotine Addiction," concluded that:

- Cigarettes and other forms of tobacco are addicting.
- Nicotine is the drug that causes this addiction.
- Quitting smoking historically has been one of the hardest addictions to break.
- The characteristics that determine nicotine addiction are similar to those that determine addiction to harder drugs such as heroin and cocaine.

To help you get more motivated to quit, I've compiled a list of lit-

Help to Quit Smoking

tle known ways your life can go up in smoke if you don't kick the habit.

From an increased risk of blindness to a faster decline in mental function, here are 10 compelling — and often surprising — reasons to stick to your resolution in 2010.

Alzheimer's Disease: Smoking Speeds Up Mental Decline

In the elderly years, the rate of mental decline is up to five times faster in smokers than in nonsmokers, according to a study of 9,200 men and women over age 65. Smoking likely puts into effect a vicious cycle of artery damage, clotting and increased risk of stroke, causing mental decline.

The bottom line: chronic tobacco use is harmful to the brain and speeds up onset of Alzheimer's disease.

Lupus: Smoking Raises Risk of Autoimmune Disease

Smoking cigarettes raises the risk of developing lupus — but quitting cuts that risk.

Systemic lupus erythematosus — known as lupus — is a chronic autoimmune disease that can cause inflammation, pain, and tissue damage throughout the body. Although some people with lupus have mild symptoms, it can become quite severe.

An Increased Risk of Impotence

Men concerned about their performance in the bedroom should stop lighting up, suggests a study that linked smoking to a man's ability to get an erection. The study of nearly 5,000 Chinese men showed that men who smoked more than a pack a day were 60% more likely to suffer erectile dysfunction, compared with men who never smoked cigarettes.

233

Overall, 15% of past and present smokers had experienced erectile dysfunction.

BLINDNESS: SMOKING RAISES RISK OF AGE-RELATED MACULAR DEGENERATION

Smokers are four times more likely to become blind because of age-related macular degeneration than those who have never smoked. But quitting can lower that risk. While all the risk factors are not fully understood, research has pointed to smoking as one major and modifiable cause.

More than a quarter of all cases of age-related macular degeneration with blindness or visual impairment are attributable to current or past exposure to smoking.

RHEUMATOID ARTHRITIS: GENETICALLY VULNERABLE SMOKERS INCREASE THEIR RISK EVEN MORE

People whose genes make them more susceptible to developing rheumatoid arthritis are even more likely to get the disease if they smoke.

In fact, certain genetically vulnerable smokers can be nearly 16 times more likely to develop the disease than nonsmokers without the same genetic profile.

SNORING: EVEN LIVING WITH A SMOKER RAISES RISK

Smoking–or living with a smoker — can cause snoring, according to a study of more than 15,000 men and women.

Habitual snoring, defined as loud and disturbing snoring at least three nights per week, affected 24% of smokers, 20% of ex-smokers, and almost 14% of people who had never smoked. The more people smoked, the more frequently they snored. Even nonsmokers were more likely to snore if they were exposed to secondhand smoke in their homes.

ACID REFLUX: HEAVY SMOKING LINKED TO HEARTBURN

People who smoke for more than 20 years are 70% more likely to have acid reflux disease than nonsmokers. Roughly one in five people suffer from heartburn or acid reflux, known medically as gastroesophageal reflux disease or GERD.

BREAST CANCER: ACTIVE SMOKING PLAYS BIGGER ROLE THAN THOUGHT

The prevalence of breast cancer among current smokers was 30% higher than the women who had never smoked — regardless of whether the nonsmokers had been exposed to secondhand or passive smoke.

Those at greatest risk: Women who started smoking before age 20, who began smoking at least five years before their first full-term pregnancy, and who had smoked for longer periods of time or smoked 20 or more cigarettes per day.

If those reasons weren't enough to motivate you to quit smoking, keep this in mind:

- Smoking is linked to certain colon cancers.
- Smoking may increase the risk of depression in young people,
- Some studies have linked smoking to thyroid disease.

Nicotine addiction is a chronic, progressive and often fatal disease. The most common treatment in the effort to assist addicted individuals in smoking cessation is nicotine replacement. This can be administered by using nicotine patches, nicotine lozenges, nicotine nasal sprays, nicotine inhalers or gum.

Natural herbal products to aid in stopping smoking can include:

- **Lobelia,** which produces effects similar to nicotine on the central nervous system and acts as a relaxant.
- **Passion Flower** promotes calmness and relaxation, which will help with the irritability you may experience.
- **Peppermint** leaf has been used for centuries for its relaxation and detoxification powers.
- **Ginger root** aids in digestion and relieves the nausea that nicotine withdrawal sometimes produces.

There are many other herbs associated with a quit smoking herbal remedy. Educate yourself on these all-natural ingredients and decide if this is a good choice for you.

If you're finally convinced you should quit, you can start right now!

SNORING

====

I'm sure just about everyone is somewhat familiar with **snoring**. Whether you call it by its slang name, "sawing logs," or its medical name, "stertor," snoring is common. You snore when something blocks the flow of air through your mouth and nose. Tissues at the top of your airway that strike each other and vibrate cause the sound.

Many adults snore, especially men.

Just about everyone snores occasionally. Even a baby or a beloved pet may snore! But snoring can affect the quantity and *quality* of your sleep. Poor sleep can lead to daytime fatigue, irritability, and increased health problems. And, if your snoring is so loud that your bed partner can't sleep, you may end up banished from the bedroom.

Snoring is the vibration of respiratory structures and the resulting sound, due to obstructed air movement during breathing while sleeping. In some cases the sound may be soft, but in other cases, it can be loud and unpleasant. Snoring during sleep may be a sign, or first alarm, of obstructive sleep apnea.

Statistics on snoring are often contradictory, but at least 30% of adults and perhaps as many as 50% of people in some demographics snore.

Although it may be upsetting to think that there could be problems at the root of you or your bed buddy's snoring, it's important to get to the bottom of it. When you do, you'll protect your health, and the intimacy of your relationship.

Age. As you reach middle age and beyond, your throat becomes narrower, and the muscle tone in your throat decreases.

- **The way you're built.** Men have narrower air passages than women and are more likely to snore. A narrow throat, a cleft palate, enlarged adenoids, and other physical attributes (which contribute to snoring) can be hereditary.
- **Nasal and sinus problems.** Blocked airways make inhalation difficult and create a vacuum in the throat, leading to snoring.
- **Being overweight or out of shape.** Fatty tissue and poor muscle tone contribute to snoring.
- **Alcohol, smoking, and medications.** Alcohol intake, smoking (or second-hand smoke), and certain medications, increase muscle relaxation leading to more snoring.
- **Sleep posture.** Sleeping flat on your back causes the flesh of your throat to relax and block the airway.

It's crucial to note to the different ways you sleep and snore. Sleep positions reveal a lot, and figuring out how you snore can reveal why you snore. When you know why you snore, you can get closer to a cure.

- Closed-mouth snoring may indicate a problem with the tongue.
- Open-mouth snoring may be related to the tissues in your throat.

Snoring

- Snoring when sleeping on back is probably mild – improved sleep habits and lifestyle changes may be effective cures.
- Snoring in *all* sleep positions can mean snoring is more severe and may require a more comprehensive treatment.

So you've tried different sleeping positions and you still suffer from noisy nights? Try the following self-help tips.

- **Lose weight.** Losing even a little bit of weight can reduce fatty tissue in the back of the throat and decrease snoring. Exercise in general can help because toning arms, legs, and abs inadvertently leads to toning muscles you don't see in the throat, which leads to less snoring.
- **Clear nasal passages.** Having a stuffy nose makes inhalation difficult and creates a vacuum in your throat, which in turn leads to snoring. You can do it naturally with a Neti pot or try nasal decongestants or nasal strips to help you breathe more easily while sleeping.
- **Quit smoking.** If you smoke, your chances of snoring are high. Smoking causes airways to be blocked by irritating the membranes in the nose and throat.
- **Establish regular sleep patterns.** Create a bedtime ritual with your partner and stick to it. Hitting the sack in a routine way together can promote better sleep and therefore minimize snoring.
- **Keep bedroom air moist** with a humidifier. Dry air can irritate membranes in the nose and throat.

- **Reposition**. Elevating your head four inches may ease breathing and encourage your tongue and jaw to move forward. (Tip: go pillow-free or try a specially designed pillow to make sure your neck muscles are not crimped).

Apart from the usual difficulties with snoring (lack of quality sleep) it can place a tremendous strain on a relationship. Even those partners who manage to put up with the snoring their health will start to suffer due to sleep deprivation which in turn can lead to daytime fatigue, irritability, raised blood pressure and so on.

One of the primary **snoring health problems** is sleep deprivation; this can affect so many areas in your day-to-day living. Your head feels soft and fuzzy, you struggle to focus on whatever you are doing, you find yourself nodding off, even worse, possibly falling asleep when you are driving, you are irritable and have a short fuse and have little patience. This can all stem from lack of sleep. You may think you have had several hours of sleep but it will not be of a deep enough sleep for your body to have a complete rest. Quality sleep is often overlooked and not placed with high enough importance and is a real cause of many *snoring health problems*. If you can get a really good night's sleep on a regular basis then the daily grind of life becomes a lot easier and you are able to deal with any issues that come your way, you become a lot more positive and you will feel a great deal healthier.

While snoring is caused by and can lead to a number of physical health problems it is also responsible for mental health and emotional issues.

For those who are not afflicted with the condition and are able to sleep without snoring, but who live with a snorer, life can become un-

Snoring

bearable. Snoring has even been cited as grounds for divorce.

It is not just the partner of a snorer who suffers. During sleeping hours, anyone who is anywhere near someone who snores will suffer. It may be other family members living in the same house; it may be neighbors in an adjoining house. With noise levels from snoring reaching the same decibel level as a jet engine–this noise can travel, even through walls.

For anyone affected by snoring, the lack of sleep over an extended period of time can have an emotional and mental impact, which is often hidden and not considered. It can be impossible for the partner of a snorer to get to sleep, let alone stay asleep.

The effects of snoring can be far reaching and are often not considered. Snoring has been known to cause marital breakdown and divorce. People have been evicted from their homes because of the noise nuisance caused by their snoring. Snoring has ended friendships between housemates. The daytime sleepiness that follows a disturbed night of inadequate sleep has caused people to lose their jobs. Snoring and the lack of sleep it causes also causes poor memory and lack of concentration.

Be proactive if you're a snorer. At least get some nasal strips. If not it can also almost ruin the perfect weekend if you're not careful...

ABOUT HAIR LOSS

=======

Hair, like every growing thing, has it's own 'cycle of life'. At any given time approximately 90 percent of the hair on your head will be in a 'growing' phase and 10 percent will be in a 'resting' phase. The growth phase lasts somewhere between two and six years while the resting phase is estimated to last anywhere from 2 – 3 months. It is after this cycle of growing and resting that a hair will die and be replaced by another new hair from the same follicle. This process begins at about the age of 10 weeks and will continue for most of your adult life – all things being equal. It is natural, therefore, to lose a certain amount of hair every day due to this natural cycle of hair growth.

About 95% of all cases of hair loss are due to what is termed Androgenetic Alopecia (commonly referred to as male pattern baldness as it occurs much more frequently in men than in women, although women can be affected by this trait also). This trait is usually inherited, although the degree to which a person can be affected by it varies from person to person.

Good strong healthy hair is, in part, reflected in the diet that we have. If your diet is lacking in the essential proteins, iron, and amino acids that are required for healthy hair, then it's only natural that your hair will suffer as a result. This may manifest itself in nothing more than dull, lifeless hair or it may result in more serious damage to the hair and the hair follicle.

Hair loss due to this trait is identifiable from the characteristic pattern of balding that a person will experience. Someone suffering from male pattern baldness will generally start to recede from the temples, the top of the head toward the back, or both. Hair will continue to recede in these areas and often result in a horseshoe type pattern of hair around a person's head. A person is programmed from birth to lose their hair. If hair loss genes are present in a person at birth, then the hair follicles on top of their head will be sensitive to the hormone dihydrotestosterone (DHT) in later life. Typically a male who experiences noticeable hair loss at an early age will tend to progress to more extensive hair loss, as they grow older.

Studies into the effects of diet and hair loss have shown that people with diets high in animal fats tend to have higher levels of testosterone released into their bloodstream and, as a result, experience higher rates of hair loss. Additionally high fat diets have also been linked to a decrease in the manufacture by the body of protein binding globulins. These globulins play an important role in neutralizing testosterone in the body until it is needed. A decrease in these globulins means a higher amount of testosterone in the blood that can be turned into hair loss inducing DHT.

So a balanced diet, rich in the right nutrients can ensure that your hair is healthy and strong and able to withstand better any genetically predisposed conditions you may have. It is interesting to observe people living in countries in Asia for example where their diet comprises large intakes of protein and nutritious vitamins and the level of hair loss that occurs in those countries compared to Western countries. The basis for their diets is vegetables, seafood, and rice for example. These items are loaded with vitamins, protein and fatty acids all of which are essential for healthy hair.

Probably the most difficult aspect of suffering from stress is identifying that you are suffering from stress in the first place. The hair and skin are normally the first places to exhibit symptoms of stress and if you are shedding hair more than usual it might be wise to examine your lifestyle and identify if undue stress could be a factor.

An increase in stress levels often manifests itself in an increase in other factors that are detrimental to healthy hair growth such as an increase in smoking, drinking coffee, and eating the wrong kinds of food. These habits go hand in hand and can often escalate if left unchecked.

Like with diet, hair loss is more than likely not the sole result of stress, but stress can certainly play a part – and like dietary deficiencies, stress-induced hair loss is reversible.

Contrary to popular belief, the gene that carries the tendency for hair loss is not inherited solely from the Mother's bloodline. The gene can also be carried over from the Father's side of the family. Additionally, just because there may be descendants from either side of the family who have exhibited hair loss, doesn't necessarily mean that future offspring will also develop the same problem. There are many factors that come into play that determine whether offspring who carry the gene for male pattern baldness will be affected by it.

About Hair Loss

Illnesses and disease, and the medications prescribed for them, can be a cause of hair loss. As has been discussed earlier, any hormonal imbalance can manifest itself in increased hair loss, so should you discover an increase in hair loss whilst on medication, consult your medical professional. Some medications are known to increase hair loss, such as medications for heart disease, high blood pressure, and arthritis to name a few.

Any kind of a disease can have some secondary effect on the scalp and hair, but some diseases, such as thyroid disease, are known to have an affect on the hair and to propagate hair loss. A thyroid test can be done by your medical professional and is nothing more than a simple blood test. Hair loss as a result of thyroid disease is reversible with correct medication for the thyroid problem. As many of the symptoms of thyroid disease are the same for many other ailments (lethargy, weight problems, hair loss, fatigue etc.), it's best to consult a medical professional if you think your hair loss may be a result of a thyroid problem – particularly before you think about spending money on any remedial products for your hair loss.

There are supplements and vitamins that can help battle hair loss. Here is a list and what they do:

- Essential fatty acids such as flaxseed oil, primrose oil and salmon oil–improve hair texture and prevent dry brittle hair
- Vitamin B complex with Vitamin B3, B5, B6–are important for the health and growth of hair
- Biotin–deficiencies have been linked to skin disorders and hair loss

- <u>Inositol</u>–vital for hair growth
- <u>Methysulfonyl-Methane (MSM)</u>–Aids with the manufacture of keratin, a protein that is the major component of hair
- <u>Vitamin C with bioflavonoids</u>–Aids in improving scalp circulation and helps with the antioxidant action in the hair follicles
- <u>Vitamin E</u>–Increases oxygen uptake, which improves circulation to the scalp and improves health and growth of hair
- <u>Zinc</u>–Stimulates hair growth by enhancing immune function
- <u>Coenzyme Q10</u>–Improves scalp circulation and increases tissue oxygenation
- <u>Kelp</u>–Needed minerals for proper hair growth
- <u>Copper</u>–Works with zinc to aid in hair growth
- <u>Grape seed extract</u>–A powerful antioxidant to protect hair follicles from free radical damage

The bottom line is that no matter how much we think we've come in terms of understanding hair loss, there is still much speculation as to its causes. Therefore it is vitally important before you take any kind of remedial action to consult with a medical professional to rule out any disease related causes that you may be unaware.

UNDERSTANDING
SCIATICA

You know what it feels like: shooting pain down your leg. You might also have tingling or numbness. Your doctor says it's sciatica, but surprisingly, sciatica isn't actually a medical condition. It's a medical term used to describe symptoms (the shooting pain, tingling, and numbness) caused by a low back condition.

Here's how it happens. Nerves extend from the brain into the arms and legs to send messages to the muscles or skin. A nerve that leaves the spine to go into the arms or legs is called a *peripheral nerve*. Peripheral nerves are bundles of millions of nerve fibers that leave the spinal cord and branch outward to other parts of the body such as muscles and skin. For example, these nerves make muscles move and enable skin sensation (feeling).

A pinched nerve in the low back usually is perceived as radiating down the leg. That means that your sciatica could be caused by a bulging disc or a herniated disc, pregnancy, spinal stenosis, a spinal tumor or spinal infection, or trauma.

Any one of those conditions can put pressure on the sciatic nerve or related nerve roots in your low back. And that pressure is what causes your pain and other symptoms.

The term sciatica describes the symptoms of leg pain and possibly tingling, numbness or weakness that originates in the low back and travels through the buttock and down the large sciatic nerve in the back of the leg.

Good news! The vast majority of people who experience sciatica get better with time (usually a few weeks or months) and find pain relief with non-surgical sciatica treatment. For others, the pain might be infrequent and irritating, but has the potential to get worse.

While sciatica can be very painful, it is rare that permanent sciatic nerve damage (tissue damage) will result.

Sciatica occurs most frequently in people between 30 and 50 years of age. Often a particular event or injury does not cause sciatica, but rather the sciatic pain over time tends to develop as a result of general wear and tear on the structures of the lower spine.

As stated earlier, in many cases, sciatica will improve and go away with time. Initial treatment usually focuses on medicines and exercises to relieve pain. You can help relieve pain by:

- Avoiding sitting (unless it is more comfortable than standing).
- Alternating lying down with short walks. Increase your walking distance, as you are able to without pain.
- Taking acetaminophen (Tylenol) or non-steroidal anti-inflammatory drugs (NSAIDs) such as ibuprofen (Advil) or naproxen (Aleve).
- Using a heating pad on a low or medium setting, or a warm

shower, for 15 to 20 minutes every 2 to 3 hours. You can also try an ice pack for 10 to 15 minutes every 2 to 3 hours. There is not strong evidence that either heat or ice will help, but you can try them to see if they help you.

Exercise like swimming strengthen the muscles that support the back without putting any strain on it or subjecting it to a sudden jolt, and can prevent and reduce the symptoms of sciatica. Yoga or Pilates can help improve the flexibility and the strength of the back muscles. Bad posture can aggravate sciatica. Taking measures to improve it can alleviate pain and swelling:

STANDING

Stand upright with a straight back and front-facing head. Weight should be balanced evenly on both feet and legs kept straight.

SITTING

Sit upright with a support, such as a cushion or rolled-up towel in the small of the back. Knees and hips should be level and feet should be flat on the floor, with the aid of a footstool if necessary.

DRIVING

As with sitting, the back should be properly supported. Correctly position wing mirrors to prevent having to twist the back. Foot controls should be squarely in front of the feet. If driving long distances, regular breaks should be taken to stretch legs.

Sleeping

Sleep on a medium-firm mattress (not too firm). The mattress should be firm enough to support the body while supporting the weight of the shoulders and buttocks, keeping the spine straight. Support the head with a pillow, but make sure the neck is not forced up at a steep angle.

Lifting and handling

To prevent injury-caused sciatica, the correct method for lifting and handling objects should be followed.

Additional treatment for sciatica depends on what is causing the nerve irritation.

If the sciatica pain is severe and has not gotten better within six to twelve weeks, it is generally reasonable to expect spine surgery to be recommended by your doctor.

Surgery speeds the resolution of pain. Two years after surgery, however, surgical and non-surgical management have about the same results; so whatever you are most comfortable with can be a valid reason to choose one or the other.

If sciatica is new to you, perhaps the most important thing to do after a days rest is to start doing gentle stretching and exercise. This may be the last thing you want to think about, particularly when it is even painful just to move. Sometimes the best way to get started is to do some gentle stretches before you get out of bed. Always ask your heath care provider what stretches or exercises are most suitable for you.

WHO'S WHO AT
TEACHING HOSPITALS?

A s always, I can count on the support of my trusted mentor from my days as a Pre-Med student at UPENN: Dr. Wesley Collier.

Each week, like clockwork, he's going to send me an article of interest, to make sure he does what he started doing for me over three decades ago. That is to make sure I don't miss out on anything that might help me on my journey.

This week, he sent me an article on something called, **The July Effect**.

That's the notion that deaths go up in July, the month that just-graduated medical residents start their new jobs, likely because of mistakes caused by inexperience.

In one recent study, researchers from the University of California at San Diego found that fatal medication errors rose 10 percent in July in U.S. counties with teaching hospitals, giving credence to what's long been known as the "July effect."

This information reminded me of some writing I did a couple of years ago, so I decided it might be useful to share some of it again.

If you've made it halfway through July without being hospitalized, and avoided the ICU on a weekend, consider yourself lucky.

More and more, many of us are finding ourselves, when we need to hospitalized, in a "teaching hospital". Many of us have had the experience of being in a hospital bed, and all of a sudden 5, 10, or sometimes 15 doctors come into the room. They surround your bed, and listen while one of them shows you off like you're a used car for sale. They point out your flaws, and your good points.

They then leave as quickly as they came in. you lie there wondering, "who were all of those people"?

You have just been "rounded" at a Teaching Hospital.

The U.S. health care system relies on teaching hospitals for the clinical education of medical students and residents. Teaching hospitals are essential "classrooms" for physicians, nurses, and other health professionals and providers.

Teaching hospitals are providers of primary care and routine patient services, as well centers for experimental, innovative and technically sophisticated services.

Additionally, teaching hospitals are special places that help the underserved and provide comprehensive and unique services for the general population. For many people, this concept of "teaching" is the notion that leads one to think, "They aren't real doctors, they are practicing on me".

A teaching hospital is a hospital which provides medical training to medical students and residents. Residents are physicians who have recently completed medical school and are in training.

Who's Who at Teaching Hospitals?

After graduating from medical school, doctors must complete a training program. This is called a "residency." During the first year of residency, a doctor is called an "intern." After the first year, interns become "residents." Both interns and residents are members of the hospital house staff. They are employed by the teaching hospital and are supervised by a hospital staff doctor.

Also called a hospital doctor or "staff" doctor, an attending physician is the doctor in charge of the patient's care. The attending is a senior doctor in general medicine or in a medical or surgical area. An attending in a teaching hospital supervises interns and residents.

Your Primary Care Doctor (also, known as your PCP) is whom you see at your regular office visit. He/She sees patients in the office setting and on "rounds", the examinations of patients in the hospital.

Many teaching hospitals have strong links with a nearby medical school.

Residency is a 3-year or more training program in a medical specialty. The first year of training after medical school is called internship, or more commonly it is called first year of residency. Much of what your doctor will learn in a chosen specialty will be learned in their residency.

After 12 years of school, 4 years of college and 4 years of medical school, there is still so much to learn. The first 20 years of school are the foundation and the tools your doctor will need to learn his/her specialty. During residency they will learn medicine by caring for patients with a variety of diseases. The more patients they care for, and the more disease and variations of disease that they see and treat, the more proficient they will become.

Here is a synopsis of different medical specialties and subspecialties and the length of their training programs (internship and residency) after medical school:

- Anesthesiology–4 years
- Dermatology–4 years
- Emergency Medicine–3-4 years
- General Surgery–5 years; Subspecialties of Surgery require an additional 1 to 4 years after the 5 year residency, they include: Vascular Surgery, Cardio-Thoracic Surgery, Pediatric Surgery, Colon and Rectal Surgery. Some surgical specialties require 1-2 years of General Surgery, then an additional 3-5 years of specialty training, they include: Neurosurgery, Orthopedic Surgery, Ophthalmology, Otolaryngology, Plastic Surgery, and Urology.
- Internal Medicine–3 years; subspecialties of Internal medicine require an additional 2-3 years after the 3 year residency, they include: Cardiology, Endocrinology, Gastroenterology, Geriatrics, Hematology, Oncology, Infectious Diseases, Nephrology, Pulmonary, Rheumatology
- Neurology–4 years
- Obstetrics and Gynecology–4 years
- Pathology–4 years
- Pediatrics–3 years; subspecialties of Pediatrics require and additional 2-3 years after the 3 year residency, they include: Pediatric Cardiology, Pediatric Endocrinology, Pediatric Gastroenterology, Pediatric Infectious Diseases, Pediatric Critical Care, Neonatology, Pediatric Nephrology, Pediatric Pulmonology, Pediatric Rheumatology

Who's Who at Teaching Hospitals?

- Psychiatry–4 years
- Radiology–4-5 years; subspecialties of Radiology require and additional 1-2 years after residency, they include: Neuroradiology, Vascular and Interventional Radiology, Pediatric Radiology.

Once all training in a specialty is completed and usually, after two or three years in practice, a physician can take Board examinations to become "Board Certified" in his or her specialty meaning they have passed an arduous test of their knowledge in the specialty. One looks for Board Certification as one measure of a physician's competence.

Most doctors are doctors of medicine (M.D.). They treat all kinds of diseases and injuries. Some doctors are doctors of osteopathic medicine (D.O.). They focus on muscles and bones. Both are able to do a residency at a teaching hospital.

So don't panic. Studies show that if you have to be in a hospital, it's safer in a teaching hospital. They have lower death rates for certain complex surgeries than non-teaching hospitals do, according to a study in the Archives of Surgery. One of the fears that many people have is that going to a teaching hospital with medical students and residents might hinder their care because the attending physicians have to teach rather than perform surgery. This study showed that perception is completely wrong. Undergoing surgery at teaching hospitals is perhaps more safe than at non-teaching hospitals because of the increased volumes of complex cases seen at these centers.

Thanks again, Dr. Collier...keep 'em coming!

A GLOSSARY OF HEALTH
REFORM TERMS

In the continuing spirit of empowering folks with information to make good decisions about their health, with changes to healthcare in the United States looming on the horizon in the upcoming years, here is a glossary of some of the more common terms you are hearing being thrown around:

Accountable Care Organization (ACO)–A network of health care providers that band together to provide the full continuum of health care services for patients. The network would receive a payment for all care provided to a patient, and would be held accountable for the quality and cost of care. New pilot programs in Medicare and Medicaid included in the health reform law would provide financial incentives for these organizations to improve quality and reduce costs by allowing them to share in any savings achieved as a result of these efforts.

Annual Benefit Limit–Insurers place a ceiling on the amount of claims they will pay in a given year for an individual. Individuals would then have to pay the full cost for any claims incurred above this ceiling during the course of the year. Beginning in 2010, annual benefit limits will be restricted and will be prohibited in 2014 under health reform.

Case Management–The process of coordinating medical care provided to patients with specific diagnoses or those with high health care needs. These functions are performed by case managers who can be physicians, nurses, or social workers.

Chronic Care Management -The coordination of both health care and supportive services to improve the health status of patients with chronic conditions, such as diabetes and asthma.

Co-ops–Private, nonprofit health organizations set up by some states to compete with private health insurers.

COBRA–Temporary continuation of health coverage at group rates available to certain former employees, retirees, spouses, and dependent children when coverage is lost due to a qualifying event, such as loss of employment. Generally, COBRA participants pay the entire premium themselves.

Coordination of benefits (COB)–A person can have more than one kind of insurance coverage, say one plan from their employer and one from their spouse's employer. In that case, the two health plans work together to coordinate which one pays first, and how much. This process is called coordination of benefits.

Diagnostic Tests–Tests and procedures ordered by a physician to determine if the patient has a certain condition or disease based upon specific signs or symptoms demonstrated by the patient. Such diagnostic tools include but are not limited to radiology, ultrasound, nuclear medicine, laboratory, pathology services or tests.

Doughnut Hole–A gap in prescription drug coverage under Medicare Part D, where beneficiaries enrolled in Part D plans pay 100% of their prescription drug costs after their total drug spending exceeds an initial coverage limit until they qualify for catastrophic coverage. Under the standard Part D benefit, Medicare covers 75% of total drug spending below the initial coverage limit ($2,830 in 2010), and 95% of spending above the catastrophic level ($6,440 in 2010). These thresholds are indexed to increase over time. The doughnut hole or coverage gap specifically refers to the range between these two levels ($3,610 in 2010) in which beneficiaries are responsible for all costs incurred for prescription drugs. The coverage gap will be gradually phased out under health reform, so that by 2020, beneficiaries will only be responsible for 25% of all prescription drug costs up to the catastrophic level.

Emergency Care–Those health care services that are provided in an emergency facility or setting after the onset of an illness or medical condition that manifests itself by symptoms of sufficient severity that without immediate medical attention could be reasonably expected by the prudent lay person, who possesses an average knowledge of health and medicine, to result in: a) placing the Member's physical and or mental health in serious jeopardy; b) serious impairment to bodily functions; or serious dysfunction of any bodily organ or part.

Employer-based health care–Refers to health plans that are offered at the workplace for employees.

Formulary–List of prescription medications covered by a health plan.

Generic Drug–A drug which is the pharmaceutical equivalent to one or more brand name drugs. Such generic drugs have been approved by the Food and Drug Administration as meeting the same standards of safety, purity, strength, dosage form, and effectiveness as the brand drug.

Government-run plan–A government-run health plan, also known as a public or single-payer plan, is modeled after Medicare, which provides individuals health care through the federal government, rather than from a private insurance company.

Grandfathered Plan–A health plan that was in place on March 23, 2010, when the health reform law was enacted, is exempt from complying with some parts of the health reform law, so long as the plan does not make significant changes to its policy, such as eliminating or reducing benefits to treat a specific disease or condition, significantly increasing cost-sharing, or reducing the employer contribution toward the premium, among others. Once a health plan makes such a change to their policy, it becomes subject to all the requirements of health reform.

Health maintenance organization (HMO)–A type of health plan that requires subscribers to receive all medical care from network providers, usually under the direction of a primary care physician (PCP)

Hospice–A facility or service that provides care for the terminally ill patient and which provides support to the family. The care, primarily for pain control and symptom relief, can be provided in the home or in an inpatient setting.

Individual mandate–In the context of health care reform, a much-discussed idea is an individual mandate, which would require all Americans to have health insurance coverage. In turn, everyone would be guaranteed coverage, regardless of age or preexisting conditions.

Inpatient–An individual who is receiving care for 24 hours or more as a registered bed patient in a hospital or other facility, where a room and board charge is made.

Long-Term Care–Services that include those needed by people to live independently in the community, such as home health and personal care, as well as services provided in institutional settings such as nursing homes. Medicaid is the primary payer for long-term care.

Medically Necessary–Procedures, treatment, supplies, equipment or services determined to be: appropriate for the symptoms, diagnosis or treatment of a medical condition, and provided for the diagnosis or direct care and treatment of the medical condition; and within generally accepted standards of good medical practice; and not primarily for the convenience of the Member or the Member's Provider; and the most appropriate procedure, treatment, supply, equipment or level of service which can be safely provided.

Outpatient Surgery–Surgical procedures performed that do not require an Inpatient admission. Such surgery can be performed in a Hospital, an Ambulatory Surgery center, or a physician office.

Preventive Care–Care rendered by a physician to promote health and prevent future health problems for a Member who does not exhibit any symptoms (for example routine physical examination, immunizations).

Pre-existing condition–If someone has shown symptoms of a health condition, or been treated for one, before their coverage begins, it is called a pre-existing condition. Usually, there is a limit to how far back a health plan can check for such conditions.

Provider network–A group of providers (such as hospitals and physicians) who agree to a pre-negotiated price for services they provide. To get that price, a patient must be covered by a particular health plan that uses that network.

Single-payer health care–In a single-payer health care system, the government collects money, primarily through tax revenue, and pays all the health care bills for its citizens.

Skilled nursing facility (SNF)–A facility licensed to provide inpatient care, including round-the-clock nursing.

Standard of care–An accepted mode of treatment for a given disease or condition.

Uninsurable–In health insurance, individuals who are "uninsurable" can't get coverage (or can get it only at higher rates) because of their medical history. It often refers to people who are already seriously ill when they apply for coverage.

Underinsured–People who have health insurance but who face out-of-pocket health care costs or limits on benefits that may affect their ability to access or pay for health care services.

Urgent Care–Services received for an unexpected episode of illness or injury requiring treatment which cannot be postponed, but is not Emergency Care. Urgent Care conditions include, but are not limited to earache, sore throat, fever not higher than 104°. Treatment of an Urgent Care condition does not require use of an emergency room at a Hospital.

Wellness Program–A health management program which incorporates the components of disease prevention, medical self-care, and health promotion. It utilizes proven health behavior techniques that focus on preventive illness and disability which respond positively to lifestyle related interventions.

GOOD HEALTHCARE: RIGHT OR PRIVILEGE

===========

"The common goal of 22 million Afro-Americans is respect as human beings, the God-given right to be a human being. Our common goal is to obtain the human rights that America has been denying us. We can never get civil rights in America until our human rights are first restored. We will never be recognized as citizens there until we are first recognized as humans."

— MALCOLM X *"Racism: the Cancer that is Destroying America"*,
in Egyptian Gazette (Aug. 25 1964) —

As America slips deeper into the bottom of the pits of despair during the current economic downturn, more and more African Americans will continue to be disproportionately represented among the uninsured, underinsured, and those joining the Medicaid rolls.

In light of the dismal response by the Federal, State, and Local governments to effectively address the Health Inequities, which impact

262

Good Healthcare: Right or Privilege

African Americans, the glaring question remains: Is good health for African Americans **right or a privilege**?

Even though they comprise a relatively small percentage of the population, as a minority group African Americans often suffer a greater percentage of incidence of many of the leading health conditions in the United States. Why is this? One potential answer to that question is health disparities. Despite the efforts to eliminate the health disparities among African Americans and the majority culture health disparities continue to exist.

The concept of health disparities is defined as differences in the occurrence, death rate, and burden of health conditions that exist among specific population groups in the United States.

The state of health for African-Americans is especially precarious. Chronic disease has an excessive impact on minority populations. Consider these facts:

- The prevalence of diabetes among African Americans is about 70% higher than among white Americans.
- Infant mortality rates are more than twice as high for African Americans as for white Americans.
- The 5-year survival rate for cancer among African Americans diagnosed for was about 44%, compared with 59% for white Americans

For African-Americans in the United States, health disparities can mean earlier deaths, decreased quality of life, loss of economic opportunities, and perceptions of injustice. For society, these disparities translate into less than optimal productivity, higher health-care costs, and social inequity.

We hold these to truths to self-evident...

Evident to whom?

Where did America go wrong? Or was it ever right?

As you would in solving any riddle, you must go back to the beginning.

Without drugging up the horrors of the "institution" called slavery, disparities in healthcare for African Americans has roots in how the medical establishment embraced an inferior view of who we were as human beings.

Benjamin Rush, a prominent Philadelphia doctor, signer of the Declaration of Independence, Dean of the Medical School at the University of Pennsylvania (and referred to as the "Father of American Psychiatry), described "Negroes" as suffering from an affliction called ***Negritude,*** which was thought to be a mild form of leprosy. The only cure for the disorder was to become white. In 1851, Dr. Samuel Cartwright, a prominent Louisiana physician and one of the leading authorities in his time on the medical care of "Negroes", identified two mental disorders peculiar to slaves. ***Drapetomia*** or the disease causing Negroes to run away, and felt that the cure, *Freedom*, however, removed all hygienic restraints, and they were no longer obedient to the laws of health, plunging into all sort of excesses and vices, leading irregular lives, and having apparently little or no control over their appetites and passions. "To sum it up, he was convinced that freedom made us nuts."

Apparently, they both failed to factor poverty, further disruption of family and kinship ties, racism, and discrimination into the high rates of insanity. As recent as the late1960s, several leading social scientists even suggested that urban violence, which most African-Americans perceived as a reaction to oppression, poverty and state-sponsored economic and physical violence against us, was actually due to "brain dysfunction, " and recommended the use of psychosurgery to prevent outbreaks of violence.

A disparity is an inequality–No if, and, or buts.

Health care should not differ by race, ethnicity, socioeconomic status, or geographic location. It is important to understand that differences in race and ethnicity (among other things) will always exist; it is wrong, however, when these differences lead to unequal healthcare.

Medical school does an excellent job of teaching the diagnosis and treatment of clinical disease but fails to prepare future physicians to incorporate psychosocial and cultural factors and overcome personal biases in the care of patients. It is reasonable to assume that the majority of healthcare provides find prejudice morally wrong, and at odds with their professional values, but healthcare providers, like other members of society, may not recognize manifestations of prejudice in their own behavior.

Approximately 12.6 % of the U.S. population – <u>38 million people</u> – identify themselves as African American. The African American population is increasing in diversity as immigrants arrive from many African and Caribbean countries. Nearly 25% of African Americans are uninsured, compared to 16% of the U.S. population. Rates of employer-based health coverage are just over 50% for employed African Americans, compared to over 70% for employed non-Hispanic whites. Medicaid covers nearly 21% of African Americans.

When African-Americans are sick and poor, they are just as en-

slaved as if the law made them so. They are not the beneficiaries of
the better health outcomes, in spite of the billions of dollars spent
on health.

A PRIMER OF MEDICAID

L ast week, during my trip to the barber shop, I had my usual health-care discussion. This time it was with a young man who made it clear how uninformed and mistaken many are on the topic of Medicaid. So, I thought, what better motivation to devote a column to this topic.

The program, known as Medicaid, became law in 1965 as a jointly funded cooperative venture between the Federal and State governments to assist states in the provision of adequate medical care to eligible needy persons. Medicaid is the largest program providing medical and health-related services to America's poorest people.

Medicaid is health insurance that helps many people who can't afford medical care pay for some or all of their medical bills. Medicaid is a health and long-term care insurance program that was established in 1965, which is also when Medicare was created.

Good health is important to everyone. If you can't afford to pay for medical care right now, Medicaid can make it possible for you to get the care that you need so that you can get healthy and stay healthy.

Medicaid is available only to people with limited income. You must meet certain requirements in order to be eligible for Medicaid. Medicaid does not pay money to you; instead, it sends payments directly to your health care providers.

The HealthChoices Program is the name of one of Pennsylvania's mandatory managed care programs for Medical Assistance recipients.

Our health-care system was actually created by accident during World War II. Because wages were frozen then, employers attracted workers with benefits such as health insurance. As a result, employer-based insurance became the foundation of the U.S. health-care system. The sad result today of that accident of history is 40 million Americans without access to basic care.

Tying health-care benefits to employers made some sense at the height of the Second Industrial Revolution, when most workers aspired to lifetime jobs with one firm. But now that the average job tenure in America is only 3 to 5 years, it no longer does. Replacing this antiquated link between employers and health insurance with a new citizen-based system could make basic health benefits universal and fully portable, both from job to job and during periods of unemployment

Medicaid was initially formulated as a medical care extension of federally funded programs providing cash income assistance for the poor, with an emphasis on dependent children and their mothers, the disabled, and the elderly. Over the years, however, Medicaid eligibility has been incrementally expanded beyond its original ties with eligibility for cash programs. Legislation in the late 1980s assured Medicaid coverage to an expanded number of low-income pregnant women, poor children, and to some Medicare beneficiaries who are not eligible for any cash assistance program. Legislative changes also focused on increased access, better quality of care, specific benefits, enhanced out-reach programs, and fewer limits on services.

In most years since its inception, Medicaid has had very rapid growth in expenditures. This rapid growth has been due primarily to the following factors:

- The increase in size of the Medicaid-covered populations as a result of Federal mandates, population growth, and the earlier economic recession. In recent years Medicaid enrollment has declined somewhat.
- The expanded coverage and utilization of services.
- The increase in the number of very old and disabled persons requiring extensive acute and/or long-term health care and various related services.
- The results of technological advances to keep a greater number of very low-birth-weight babies and other critically ill or severely injured persons alive and in need of continued extensive and very costly care.
- The increase in drug costs and the availability of new expensive drugs.
- Good health is important to everyone. If you can't afford to pay for medical care right now, Medicaid can make it possible for you to get the care that you need so that you can get healthy – and stay healthy.

Medicaid operates as a vendor payment program. States may pay health care providers directly on a fee-for-service basis, or States may pay for Medicaid services through various prepayment arrangements, such as health maintenance organizations (HMOs). Within Federally imposed upper limits and specific restrictions, each State for the most part has broad discretion in determining the payment methodology and payment rate for services. Generally, payment rates must be sufficient to enlist enough providers so that covered services are available at least to the extent that comparable care and services are available to the general population within that geographic area. Providers participating in Medicaid must accept Medicaid payment rates as payment in full. States must make additional payments to qualified hospitals that provide inpatient services to a disproportionate number of Medicaid beneficiaries and/or to other low-income or uninsured persons under what is known as the "disproportionate share hospital" (DSH) adjustment.

The changes to the Medicaid program under Heath Reform, the Patient Protection and Affordability Care Act (PPACA) significantly expand Medicaid coverage for adults.

Advocates need to be aware, that states usually follow some basic rules of thumb for reducing Medicaid expenditures:

1. Reduce or eliminate staff and impose travel and hiring freezes.
2. Cut provider reimbursement rates.
3. Increase or start copayments and cut the amount, duration, and scope of optional benefits.
4. Drop optional services such as vision, dental, chiropractic, and podiatric care.
5. Tighten eligibility criteria and limits.

When advocates know the basic strategies and look into how

their state responded in the past, they then need to realize that opposing one cut in Medicaid could result in an undesirable cut of another Medicaid benefit.

Advocates should weigh the pros and cons of increasing revenues to reinstate Medicaid costs. It makes sense to increase the cigarette tax to support health and human services rather than cut health care. It also is logical to advocate spending rainy day or surplus funds instead of cutting Medicaid benefits and losing federal matching funds.

Medicaid recipients in Pennsylvania could have trouble getting care next year because of the state's fiscal woes, according to health plan executives across the state.

Medical Assistance is Pennsylvania's version of the state/federal Medicaid program, which provides health insurance to the poor and disabled. As of 2009, 36% of Pennsylvanians are at or below the Federal poverty Level. That means almost 4 out of every 10 people in Pennsylvania are eligible for Medicaid!

With the recently passed Healthcare Reform, for the first time, single adults who are not disabled, who are not elderly, would be guaranteed access to the Medicaid program if their income was below a certain level. This is a fundamental change in the way this country has approached the Medicaid program.

In many ways, the fate of health care reform depends on the fate of Medicaid.

"EQUITY" IN HEALTHCARE
REFORM

====================

The U.S. health system is the most expensive in the world, but comparative analyses consistently show the United States underperforms relative to other countries on most dimensions of performance. Most U.S. residents want a society in which all persons live long, healthy lives; however, that vision is yet to be realized fully, even in the face of the recent Health Reform legislation.

In spite of the fact that The United Nations has declared 2011 "The International Year for People of African Descent", African Americans are still experiencing inequity and disparities in health care.

According to the organizations' website, "The Year aims at strengthening national actions and regional and international cooperation for the benefit of people of African descent in relation to their full enjoyment of economic, cultural, social, civil and political rights, their participation and integration in all political, economic, social and cultural aspects of society, and the promotion of a greater knowledge of and respect for their diverse heritage and culture."

Health equity is the right of all members of society to achieve the best possible health and to not have their health negatively affected by avoidable, unfair, and unjust policies or conditions within the system in which they live. However, not everyone has a voice at the table—especially underrepresented groups who are socioeconomically disadvantaged or who have been victims of historical injustices. Inequitable distribution of or access to social, economic, and health resources can affect a groups' attitude, behavior and health outcomes.

The socioeconomic circumstances of persons and the places where they live and work strongly influence their health. In the United States, as elsewhere, the risk for mortality, morbidity, unhealthy behaviors, reduced access to health care, and poor quality of care increases with decreasing socioeconomic circumstances.

Health equity is achieved when every person has the opportunity to "attain his or her full health potential" and no one is "disadvantaged from achieving this potential because of social position or other socially determined circumstances." Health inequities are reflected in differences in length of life; quality of life; rates of disease, disability, and death; severity of disease; and access to treatment.

Social determinants of health are the key factors in the health status gap between blacks and whites. Social determinants of health are the social, economic and political forces under which people live that affect their health. Social determinants include wealth/income, education, physical environment, health care, housing, employment, stress and racism/discrimination. In fact, for blacks racism is a key factor. Even when economics are controlled, blacks have poorer health. That is, middle-class blacks have poorer health than middle-class whites. In fact, middle-class whites live 10 years longer than middle-class blacks. The stress of living in a racialized discriminatory society accounts for these racial health disparities.

The single biggest threat to stemming rising costs, that heath reform is supposed to address, is the uncontrolled increase in chronic illnesses like diabetes and asthma, and related conditions such as obesity. We as a nation must give chronic diseases the attention they demand.

Chronic diseases are characterized by often being permanent; rarely cured; and needing long-term care. Nearly one in two Americans (133 million) has a chronic medical condition of one kind or another. The leading chronic diseases in developed countries include arthritis, cardiovascular disease such as heart attacks and stroke, cancer such as breast and colon cancer, diabetes, epilepsy and seizures, obesity, and oral health problems.

The real tragedy is that many of the 1.7 million deaths among Americans from chronic diseases each year are in large part preventable. Chronic diseases impose an enormous financial and societal burden on the United States.

According to the Centers for Disease Control and Prevention (CDC), chronic diseases today account for 70% of the deaths of all Americans and 75% of this country's annual health care costs. Unless we take steps now to deal effectively with chronic diseases, our nation is headed for a serious financial and quality-of-life crisis. Among the contributing factors to this crisis are the aging of our population; increases in obesity, particularly among adolescents; and the tragedy of tobacco addiction.

They represent 75 percent of the $2.2 trillion spent on health care in the U.S. in 2007–and are the primary driver of rising costs. In tax-payer-funded programs such as Medicare and Medicaid, the proportions are even higher: 96% and 83%, respectively.

In 1900, the top three causes of death in the United States were pneumonia/influenza, tuberculosis, and diarrhea. Communicable diseases accounted for about 60 percent of all deaths. In 1900, heart disease and cancer were ranked number four and eight respectively. Since the 1940s, most deaths in the United States have resulted from heart disease, cancer, and other degenerative diseases. And, by the late 1990s, degenerative diseases accounted for more than 60 percent of all deaths.

Scientific evidence suggests that it is possible that maintaining a healthy lifestyle can prevent and control chronic disease. Major risk factors that have been proven to contribute to chronic diseases are unhealthy diets, lack of physical activity, and smoking.

Taking steps to reduce risk factors throughout life can have a massive impact on the control of chronic disease. For instance, 80% of cases of coronary heart disease, 90% of cases of type 2 diabetes, and about one-third of cancers could be avoided by elimination of certain risk factors.

Four healthy lifestyle factors can help keep the most common and deadly chronic diseases at bay. The four healthy lifestyle factors are never smoking, maintaining a healthy weight, exercising regularly and following a healthy diet.

Socio-economic & environmental factors that influence to health outcomes:

- Education
- Employment

- Family structure
- Housing and home environment
- History
- Community infrastructure

The Centers for Disease Control and Prevention (CDC) has identified the following behaviors that put people at risk for chronic disease and premature death:

- Smoking and other tobacco use
- High-fat, low fiber diet
- Physically inactive
- Lack of preventative health services (cancer screenings, cholesterol checks, blood pressure checks)

Because of the increasing burden of chronic diseases, the United States faces a potential financial and health care crisis of unparalleled proportion. And while the human cost is enormous, the economic cost also is great. The cost of treating these conditions — without even taking into consideration the many secondary health problems they cause — totaled $277 billion in 2003, and continues to climb. These conditions also reduce productivity at the workplace, as ill employees and their caregivers are often forced either to miss work days (absenteeism) or to show up but not perform well. The impact of lost workdays and lower employee productivity resulted in an annual economic loss in the United States of over $1 trillion in 2003. Chronic disease prevention is a beneficial method of cost reduction in health care services. For example, each dollar spent on school-based tobacco, drug, alcohol, and sexuality education programs provides a savings of $14 in health care costs.

It is incumbent upon us, in spite of what they are calling "Health Reform" to join in ensuring that our nation's political leaders and the citizens they represent better understand the profound burden of chronic disease and the positive efforts that need to be taken now to reduce that burden. Our nation, our communities, and our families deserve no less.

CLINICAL TRIALS

===================

C linical trials are a vital and necessary part of America's medical research system. They have proven to be the best mechanism for testing potential drugs and separating the ones that work from the ones that are ineffective or potentially harmful.

It usually takes 12–15 years for a new compound to be approved as a medicine in the United States. On average, it costs $800 million for a pharmaceutical company to develop a new medicine. Typically, a pharmaceutical company recoups its development costs for only three of ten medicines.

Before 1938, manufacturers could market a drug without submitting any information to the FDA or any other agency; the Federal Food, Drug and Cosmetic Act (FD&C Act) of 1938 was passed when over 100 children died from taking a sulfa drug that had not been tested in people.

One of the major events that brought the issue of clinical trials to the public was the revelation of the Tuskegee Syphilis Study. The United States Public Health Service conducted the study. The Tuskegee study began in 1932 and continued till 1972, when it was revealed to the public. The purpose of the study was to examine the long-term affects of syphilis. The subjects of the study were 400 African American males, who were primarily poor sharecroppers. These men all had syphilis, but were unaware of it. They were also unaware of the true nature of the experiment. The most horrifying aspect of the experiment was in the 1950's penicillin was proved to be effective at curing syphilis. The researchers did not treat the syphilis and even prevented other doctors who saw the participants from treating the syphilis. As many as one hundred men may have died from complications from their untreated syphilis. The study was revealed in 1972 by a newspaper article shocked the country and caused the project to be shut down. It wasn't until 1997 that President Clinton formally apologized for the study.

Many of the early advances in medicine were made at the expense of many marginal groups such as asylum inmates and prisoners. These test subjects were involved in these clinical trials without being informed, or even asked.

Informed consent is one of the most important "safety nets" in clinical trials. Doctors are obligated to make sure that a patient understands the risks and benefits of any medical procedure. Requiring informed consent protects many marginal groups from being forced to participate in medical studies without understanding the risks involved. Medical advances should not require some people to sacrifice their health and rights for the good of all. Informed consent is a key instrument in protecting these rights.

At the start of the four "Phase" clinical drug trial, developers concentrate on the tolerability of a new drug. These Phase I studies are usually carried out on a small number (20–100) of healthy volunteers. The aim of Phase II studies, which include 100 to 500 patients, is to determine whether the new drug is effective in the disease for which it is intended and what its potential side effects are. Phase II studies also serve to determine the dosage range, i.e. the highest tolerable and lowest effective doses, for the subsequent large-scale Phase III studies.

To this end, the patients are divided into two study groups. One patient group (the drug group) receives the drug being tested, while the other (the control group) receives a standard medication or placebo (placebo group). A placebo is a dummy pill, tablet, capsule, or solution that is identical in color and taste to the drug but contains no active ingredient.

For ethical reasons, in the case of severe and life-threatening diseases such as cancer and Aids, both groups continue to take their standard medications as well as the new drug or placebo.

Most clinical drug trials are based on a "blind" design, i.e. the patients are unaware which group they have been assigned to. In many cases, moreover, neither the patients nor the developers know who is receiving the test drug. Such trials are referred to as double-blind studies.

Phase III studies are carried out on large groups of patients (1,000 to 5,000) for whom the new drug is ultimately intended. The inclusion criteria that determine which patients can be enrolled in the study are often less stringent than in Phase II. Patients who differ in terms of gender, age, ethnic origin, lifestyle, diet, and state of health are randomly selected.

In order to recruit the large number of voluntary patients required, the studies are usually organized on at a number of hospitals and medical practices.

Clinical Trials

Once approval has been granted by the regulatory authorities, the pharmaceutical company is allowed to market the drug. Even then, however, the manufacturer has to submit to the regulatory authorities a precisely scheduled series of reports (phase IV) to document very rare side effects of the drug which occur in, say, only out one of 20,000 cases and which can therefore escape notice even in the Phase III trials.

As beneficial as clinical trials are, there are concerns. In all things you must "follow the money".

Costing upwards of a half billion dollars, and taking up to ten years before any return on investment, the stakes are indeed high. Private corporations, not the government, have been the largest sponsors of pharmaceutical research in both the United States in the last twenty years.

While doctors have a right to be reasonably remunerated for the work they perform, inappropriate remuneration raises the possibilities of:

- Erosion of the patient's informed consent;
- Enrolment of ineligible subjects or subjects on the margins of eligibility;
- A coercive enrollment environment, e.g., patients agreeing to be subjects simply because they fear losing the caregiver if they say 'no'; and
- Doctors, under pressure to increase their income, being inclined to perform research that they are not qualified to do.

Never feel pressured into joining a clinical trial. If your questions are not fully answered by the research nurse or doctor at the outset, discuss the benefits and risks of participating with your family doctor before signing a consent form. If you have any concerns during the trial, contact the clinician in charge or the head of the institution's ethics committee that approved the trial. (You should have been given the committee's telephone number). If the ethical approval was by a for-profit company, seek advice from your family physician as to whether it's advisable to continue in the trial. You can withdraw from the study at any time for whatever reason. If you plan to stop participating, you might let the research team know why you are leaving the study, although you are not required to explain your decision for withdrawing to anyone.

Here are some other questions to keep in mind about clinical trials: Do they offer false hope? Do enough people take part? Is it better or worse if a study is funded by a large pharmaceutical company? I don't think much has been written about this topic, but it's time we started talking... and thinking.

AGE IS JUST A NUMBER

W̶e live in a world that is obsessed with looking young and beautiful. Faced with loss of youth, many of us feel profound fear, loneliness, and regret—which leads to the depressing idea that the best years of our lives are behind us.

Aging is something we all do but understand very little. We could list things that change as we age (memory loss, wrinkles, muscles loss, balance trouble, etc.) but no one really understands what aging is, why it happens or how to stop it.

Most people are scared, indeed, terrified of old age because they feel that aging is characterized by a progressive loss of essential body functions that they have learnt to take for granted over the years; for instance, loss of vision, hearing, teeth, memory, intelligence, sexual drive, muscle strength and vigor. However, it needs to be emphasized that you can become old healthily; remember that old age does not necessarily mean progressive deterioration or susceptibility to a plethora of ailments!

Fortunately, aging doesn't have to be a downhill slides and gaining adequate knowledge about changing body patterns over time can help you age the healthy way. Older people have the reputation of being more mature, experienced and thoughtful. Whether or not you become wiser as you grow older, you are likely to become farsighted for sure! Farsightedness (presbyopia), one example of aging, is a change in vision that's a normal part of aging. A gradual hardening of the eye's lens, which impairs your ability to see up close, causes it. Your optometrist may recommend a pair of non-prescription reading glasses or prescribe bifocals for you.

Aging is nothing more than the natural wear and tear of the body's component parts. It's inevitable, and endlessly intriguing. While many age-related changes cannot be prevented, a lifestyle that includes exercise and a well-balanced diet will slow or minimize many problems related to aging.

As we age, our body's organs and other systems make changes. These changes alter our susceptibility to various diseases. Researchers are just beginning to understand the processes that cause changes over time in our body systems. Understanding these processes is important because many of the effects of aging are first noticed in our body systems. Here is a brief overview of how some body systems age:

- **Heart Aging:** The heart muscle thickens with age as a response to the thickening of the arteries. This thicker heart has a lower maximum pumping rate.
- **Immune System Aging:** T cells take longer to replenish in older people and their ability to function declines.
- **Arteries and Aging:** Arteries usually to stiffen with age, making it more difficult for the heart to pump blood through them.

- **Lung Aging:** The maximum capacity of the lungs may decrease as much as 40 percent between ages 20 and 70.

- **Brain Aging:** As the brain ages, some of the connections between neurons seem to be reduced or less efficient. This is not yet well understood.

- **Kidney Aging:** The kidneys become less efficient at cleaning waste from the body.

- **Bladder Aging:** The total capacity of the bladder declines and tissues may atrophy, causing incontinence.

- **Body Fat and Aging:** Body fat increases until middle age and then weight typically begins to decrease. The body fat also moves deeper in the body as we age.

- **Muscle Aging:** Muscle tone declines about 22 percent by age 70, though exercise can slow this decline.

- **Bone Aging:** Starting at age 35, our bones begin to lose density. Walking, running and resistance training can slow this process.

- **Sight and Aging:** Starting in the 40s, difficulty seeing close detail may begin.

- **Hearing and Aging:** As people age, the ability to hear high frequencies declines.

Staying active is a terrific way to stave off the negative effects of aging because it helps your body maintain, improve and even repair itself. Physical activity increases flexibility, lowers blood pressure, strengthens bones, slows down the process of osteoporosis, and promotes weight loss. The remarkable aspect about getting fit is that it's never too late to start. Fifteen to 30 minutes of exercise, with a warm-up and a cool-down, three or four times a week, would be ideal. Remember to start out slowly, exercising for about five to ten minutes twice a week, and gradually build up to a higher level of activity. Choose an activity that you'll enjoy, and try to get a friend to accompany you. Brisk walking, swimming and yoga are just a few of the options. Before starting your regular exercise regimen, please check with your doctor about possible complications or risks.

Never think of age as being anything but just a number. There are some things in life we have no control over, such as when we were born. Age is no more than a circumstantial detail, like the color of your eyes, or the names of your parents; it does **not** define who you are. Aging is inevitable, growing old is avoidable. Expressed differently, one is never too young to be old or eve die, but one is never so aged as to become old.

Illness and aging need not go hand in hand. If you take good care of your body in the 'morning', it will take good care of you in the 'evening' of your life.

Don't give up the ship. Even if you're pretty sure you've taken less than the best care of the body you were given, it isn't too late to fix some things, according to the medical experts. Talk to a nutritionist–you'll be fascinated by how simple it is to make small changes with big results. Start moving about more–exercise can be fun. You can count everyday activities as exercise. Energetic house cleaning, walking up and down stairs, swimming, and so forth all count. You've heard the recent advice–park your car farther from the store. Use stairs, not elevators. Get up from the couch or computer every hour and do something active.

Develop a good relationship with a doctor you trust and see that doctor regularly. Talk over things that concern you. Keep an eye on your partner or spouse and ask them to monitor your health visually, too.

Read a lot–keep up to date on the latest health information and take the steps that seem viable or rational to your situation. You live in an excellent time–medication, therapies, science and research are increasing life expectancies almost daily. Do your part and make the most of what you have.

It's never too late to adopt a healthy lifestyle. You can't stop the aging process, but you can minimize the impact by making healthy lifestyle choices.

CAREGIVING FOR
A LOVED ONE

$=$

A growing issue for many of us is suddenly finding ourselves in the role of Caregiver, without a clue as to how to function best. While the primary responsibility for medical care rests between the physician and patient, you may be assisting with medication management, and helping your care receiver to understand his or her medical care.

If you are having difficulty affording medication, and cannot fill the prescription, let your physician know before you leave his/her office.

Ask the physician what is the name of the drug? Brand name? Generic name? What is the drug for? What symptoms will it treat? Are there any side effects to be alert for? Should the medication be taken with food? Are there foods, activities, or drugs that should be avoided while taking the medication? What should be done if a dose is missed?

It is recommended that all individuals use **one pharmacy** so that the professional pharmacist can assist in your medication management.

Keep your medicine in its original bottle.

Know what you are taking. Many similar medications have different brand or generic names.

Make sure your physician knows **ALL** of the medications you use. This includes over-the-counter medicines, vitamins, minerals, and herbal remedies. Throw out old medication.

As one's memory fades, the caregiving challenge begins. It is important to remember at this time that people do not consist of memory alone. They have feelings, will, sensibility, and moral being. Diseases that cause memory loss, including Alzheimer's disease and other Dementia diseases, Parkinson's disease, and strokes, have a variety of symptoms that can overwhelm family caregivers.

If the individual is not feeling well, has pain, is coming down with a cold, has a medication reaction, or an infection, you will probably see a sudden onset of problematic behaviors and confusion that does not go away with rest. If this happens, and the individual does not improve in an hour, complains of pain, shortness of breath, is bleeding, or vomiting, the individual needs to see the doctor as soon as possible.

Some common problems to consider:

- Has the individual been drinking at least one and a half quarts of liquid each day?
- Are they urinating frequently?
- Does their urine smell strong? Urinary tract infections are very common causes of agitation.
- Does the person have arthritis or another painful condition?
- Is the individual on his/her feet all day?
- Does the individual "hold" or protect a part of his/her body?

Even though the individual may not complain of pain, it may be there. If the individual begins to moan, yell, or scream, suspect that he/she might be in pain.

- Worry about constipation. Make sure the individual receives adequate fiber in his/her diet. Severe constipation is a common cause of fever and a mild fever in an aged person can cause agitation, confusion, lethargy.

- Have the individual's prescriptions, over-the-counter medications, vitamins, and herbal preparations checked and reviewed by the doctor regularly.

- Avoid alcohol intake as it can worsen memory permanently. Many people with memory loss over-react to alcohol.

The doctor is your most valuable resource. He/she should be chosen carefully. The doctor you choose should be able to meet both the care receiver's needs and yours, too. You may want to consider:

- Does the doctor have the training and background that meets the needs of the care receiver?

- Does the doctor have privileges at the hospital that is closest to your home? If the care receiver becomes ill, what are his/her emergency procedures?

- Does the doctor give you an opportunity to ask questions? Does he/she encourage you to ask questions? Does he/she answer questions in a clear and understanding way?

- Does the doctor treat both you and the care receiver with dignity and respect?

- Does the doctor consider you a part of the treatment team?
- Does the doctor offer written information on a particular diagnosis or condition?
- Will the doctor provide comprehensive care for both you and the care receiver?
- Does the doctor or someone else in the office speak the primary language that you (and the care receiver) are most comfortable with?
- Who covers for the doctor when he/she is not available?
- How long do you have to wait to get a routine appointment?
- How long do you and the care receiver need to wait in the office before seeing the doctor? (This is important if the care receiver is diagnosed with dementia, and becomes anxious in different surroundings).
- Will the office call and remind you about appointments?
- What happens when my care receiver has an emergency?
- Can you call and get advice over the phone for common medical problems and health care concerns?
- Does the doctor provide you with choices as to medications and treatment options?
- Does the doctor explain the purpose of diagnostic testing requested? He/she should be able to tell you why the test is requested, what he/she will learn from the test, any risk associated with the test, and why the test is justified.

Never be embarrassed to discuss **ANY** topic with the doctor. Lastly, remember the doctor you choose is a human being, with enormous responsibilities. Be polite, and value each other.

As for how you treat the person receiving the care, treat them well and with respect. My Grandpapa always used to say; "You've got to be careful because you never know who will bring **you** a glass of water in the morning".

PLANNING FOR THE "LAST GOODBYE"

Here in America, our culture, tells us that we should fight hard against age, illness and death. And holding on to life, to our loved ones, is indeed a basic human instinct. However, as the end of life approaches, letting go" may not feel like the right thing to do.

Americans are a people who plan. We plan everything: our schedules, our careers and work projects, our weddings and vacations, our retirements. Many of us plan for the disposition of our estates after we die. The one area that most of us avoid planning is the end of our life. Yet, if we don't plan, if we don't at least think about it and share our ideas with those we love, others take over at the very time when we are most vulnerable, most in need of understanding and comfort, and most longing for dignity.

Most people do not die traumatically. Instead, the last days of their lives are spent in a hospital, nursing home, or in their own home. In your advance directive (see below), you can state your preferences about where you wish to be in the event of terminal illness or during the process of dying. If you choose to be at home, many home care options are available, including home health and custodial care.

Advance directives are written instructions that communicate your wishes about the care and treatment you want to receive if you reach the point where you can no longer speak for yourself. Medicare and Medicaid *require* that health care facilities that receive payments from them provide patients with written information concerning the right to accept or refuse treatment and to prepare advance directives. Every state now recognizes advance directives, but the laws governing directives vary from state to state.

Probably the most commonly used form of advance directive is the *durable power of attorney for health* care (or Health Care Proxy). This is a document in which you appoint someone else to make medical treatment decisions for you if you cannot make them for yourself. This is certainly a wise move to make, because if you do not name a proxy or agent, the likelihood of needing a court-appointed guardian (like the hospital itself) grows greater, especially if there is disagreement regarding your treatment among your family and doctors.

It is wise to have an advance directive so that medical personnel and your loved ones will know what care and services you prefer and what treatment you would refuse, in the event that you are unable communicate your wishes. You also can designate the person or more than one person who you would like to make decisions on your behalf. In a surprising number of families, there is disagreement over what a very ill relative would prefer. The advance directive makes your wishes clear. An advance directive can express **both** what you want and don't want.

Planning for the "Last Goodbye"

Even if you do not want treatment to cure you, you should always be kept reasonably pain free and comfortable.

It's best to think of Advance Health Care Directives as a work in progress. Circumstances can change, as can your values and opinions about how you would best like your future health care needs to be met. Directives can be revoked or replaced at any time as long as you are capable of making your own decisions. It is recommended that you review your documents every few years or after important life changes and revise your directives to ensure that they continue to accurately reflect your situation and wishes.

Re-examine your health care wishes every few years or whenever any of the "Five D's" occur:

- **Decade** – when you start each new decade of your life.
- **Death** – whenever you experience the death of a loved one.
- **Divorce** – when you experience a divorce or other major family change.
- **Diagnosis** – when you are diagnosed with a serious health condition.
- **Decline** – when you experience a significant decline or deterioration of an existing health condition, especially when it diminishes your ability to live independently.

Another form or method of instruction available to you is a Do Not Resuscitate or DNR order, which instructs medical personnel, including emergency medical personnel, not to use resuscitative measures. A do-not-resuscitate (DNR) order tells medical professionals not to perform CPR. This means that doctors, nurses and emergency medical personnel will not attempt emergency CPR if the patient's breathing or heartbeat stops.

DNR orders may be written for patients in a hospital or nursing home, or for patients at home. Hospital DNR orders tell the medical staff not to revive the patient if cardiac arrest occurs. If the patient is in a nursing home or at home, a DNR order tells the staff and emergency medical personnel not to perform emergency resuscitation and not to transfer the patient to a hospital for CPR.

Ask your doctor for a time when you can go over your ideas and questions about end-of-life treatment and medical decisions. Tell him or her you want guidance in preparing advance directives. If you are already ill, ask your doctor what you might expect to happen when you begin to feel worse. Let him or her know how much information you wish to receive about your illness, prognosis, care options, and hospice programs.

Medical advances make it possible to keep a person alive who, in former times, would have died more quickly from the serious nature of their illness, injury or infection. This has set the stage for ethical and legal controversy about the patient's rights, the family's rights and the medical profession's proper role.

Each American has the constitutional right, established by a Supreme Court decision, to request that medical treatment be withdrawn or withheld. The right remains valid even if you become incapacitated. Doctors can always refuse to comply with your wishes if they have an objection based on their own religious beliefs, for example, or consider your wishes medically inappropriate. However, they may have an obligation to transfer you to another healthcare provider who will comply with your wishes.

Questions you should ask your doctor if you are diagnosed with a terminal illness:

- Tell me straight: How long do I realistically have?
- Realistically, what can I expect in terms of symptoms and process?
- What if I go Route A or Route B?
- What do you think I should do and why?

All of these questions may sound very difficult to discuss now, when the time for decisions is still in the future. However, they are harder to discuss when someone is really sick, emotions are high, and decisions must be made quickly.

It is true that more older, rather than younger, people use advance directives, but every adult should have one. Younger adults actually have more at stake, because, if stricken by serious disease or accident, medical technology may keep them alive but insentient for decades. Some of the most well-known "right to die" cases arose from the experiences of young people (e.g., Karen Ann Quinlan, Terri Schiavo) incapacitated by tragic illnesses or car accidents and maintained on life support.

Looking at all the information available and making the best decision you can, will give you peace of mind, and the comforting awareness that you did what was right as you knew it.

Glenn Ellis
Strategies for Well-Being, LLC
Post Office Box 5331
Yeadon, Pennsylvania 19050
USA
info@glennellis.com
www.glennellis.com

Made in the USA
Middletown, DE
12 January 2018